THE BODY MYTH

Also by Milli Hill

The Positive Birth Book
Give Birth Like a Feminist
My Period
Ultra-Processed Women

THE BODY MYTH

Milli Hill

HQ

ONE PLACE. MANY STORIES

HQ
An imprint of HarperCollins*Publishers* Ltd
1 London Bridge Street
London SE1 9GF

www.harpercollins.co.uk

HarperCollins*Publishers*
Macken House, 39/40 Mayor Street Upper,
Dublin 1, D01 C9W8, Ireland

This edition 2026

1
First published in Great Britain by HQ,
an imprint of HarperCollins*Publishers* Ltd 2026

A catalogue record for this book is available from the British Library.

HB ISBN: 978-0-00-859900-3
TPB ISBN: 978-0-00-867344-4

This book is set in 10.7/15.5 pt. Sabon by Type-it AS, Norway

Printed and bound in the UK using 100% Renewable
Electricity by CPI Group (UK) Ltd

FSC
www.fsc.org
MIX
Paper | Supporting responsible forestry
FSC® C013604

To my mum, Pauline Hill, and the women of our shared red thread, past and future.

Contents

Let Me Tell You a Story...

This is a book about body myths – the stories we tell about life in the female body – and how these stories make us feel.

It's also a book about how brilliant that female body is.

We know the negatives – some of them are neatly embedded in our daily thoughts, giving us their unwanted opinions each time we walk across a crowded room or change our tampon or have sex or look in the mirror. Others are increasingly well documented: for example, the fact that women's bodies have been left out of scientific research and sidelined in the way the world around us has been designed. We know that the male body has historically been seen as the 'default' or 'best' or, at the very least, 'standard' body, and the female as a slightly unreliable, complex and occasionally somewhat leaky second edition. In our collective consciousness, man came first and woman was hastily cobbled together out of a spare bit of him when he got lonely. But what if we changed that story? This book will take you on a journey through some of the familiar negatives, but only in order to repeatedly challenge them and offer you, the reader, a sort of 'giant reframe'.

The female body has had a consistently bad press for much of recorded time. To unpick this, it's interesting to ask who has been telling, and continues to tell, this story. This book appears in the midst of what can only be described as a patriarchal backlash, as women are encouraged into regressive stereotypes, reproductive rights are rolled back, male violence against women and girls remains unchecked, and attempts at body positivity are challenged by porn and by a culture that says, 'Don't like what you see? There's a procedure / filter / drug for that.' The female body continues to be a battleground; commodified, mistreated, cut and adapted, controlled, pathologised, silenced, bought and sold. Against this backdrop, repeated stories of female bodily inadequacy are a gift to the patriarchal status quo, characterising us as inherently lesser, unreliable, weak and in need of management, adaptation and guidance.

Most people are now familiar with concepts from medical history such as 'hysteria', in which the womb goes on an unchaperoned wander around the body, causing all manner of physical and psychological disorders and making us wholly unsuitable for public office. It's easy to laugh about this now, but we still live in a world where the ramifications of characterising women as physically and mentally inferior, and therefore undeserving of the same rights and opportunities as men, continue to be felt. On the basis of our sex, we are still paid less, given less positions of power, our sexuality and appearance controlled and judged, our bodies exploited and legislated over. It's a power game, in which the female body is not properly researched, while at the same time women suffer unexplained chronic health conditions that actually do impact on their ability to participate in the world, thus reinforcing the myth of their inadequacy. While it may be difficult to measure the impact of this, what we can quantify more clearly is how much money there is to be made from continuing to maintain that women's bodies don't quite measure up. Wherever there is a story being told of female inadequacy, there is always someone monetising it, whether this is mainstream or alternative medicine, cosmetic surgeons, formula milk companies or innovative tech firms offering futuristic solutions to an age-old problem.

Against this backdrop, it is quietly subversive to ask the question: what is good about life in a female body? Even the idea of 'body positivity', which currently struggles against the tide in a world of TikTok filters and Ozempic, is centred around how we *look* rather than what our bodies *do*. In celebrating bodies that don't conform to rigid beauty standards, the focus remains on women's outer appearance and unwittingly plays into centuries of emphasis on the female form as passive, decorative and there for the pleasure of others, rather than as potent, active, independent and strong. It's time for a new kind of body positivity, which doesn't just celebrate the female body when it's in the still life of a photograph or being appraised as a mirror reflection, but also takes pride in it when it's in action – bleeding, birthing, lactating – doing any of the mind-blowingly powerful things it – and only it – can actually *do*.

My thoughts about this book developed out of the work around 'birth positivity' that I've been involved in for a decade or so, as founder of the Positive Birth Movement and the author of two books about reclaiming childbirth as an active, powerful experience, and also from the feedback I received about my third book, *My Period*, which is aimed at pre-teen girls and is all about puberty and menstruation. A lot of the messages I've had about that book have not been from young readers, but from their mums, along the lines of: 'I wish I'd had this book when I was growing up!' or, 'Why did nobody teach me this at school!' and, 'It's made me see my body completely differently!' I started to connect the dots between positive birth and positive puberty, and realise that they are both counterpoints to a lifetime of negative messaging that women receive about their body's abilities. From puberty all the way through to menopause, women are taught to feel shame, doubt and fear about their bodies, and to view being female as somehow the short straw.

This lie we are all taught in a multitude of ways does not bear much scrutiny. As you will find in this book, every single story of shame, doubt and fear can be quite easily wiped away, like a painting restorer carefully removing a few centuries of muck and varnish to reveal the hidden masterpiece beneath. Wherever there is a negative story about the female body, this is a clue in itself and a sign to look deeper. Instead of accepting it on surface value, we need to begin wiping away the layers. Almost always the same picture will be revealed: women are not weak or defective at all, they are powerful. Rather than being a 'curse', life in a female body, with all its unique abilities, is actually a gift.

This book is for you whether you love being female, feel ambivalent towards it or frequently wish for a different lot in life. You are most welcome to read it if you are male, but, in all honesty, I wrote it with women at the forefront of my mind, and it is the female psyche that I hope shifts as a result of this book's existence. One of the most simple and powerful lessons I learned, through my former career as a therapist, and through having therapy myself, was that you only ever have the power to change yourself. Frustration often comes in life as a result of the behaviour, thoughts or attitudes of others – over which we are unfortunately powerless. However, if we change ourselves – which is infinitely possible – then those around us will inevitably be nudged into change as a result. I truly believe that if women begin to think differently about themselves and their bodies, then this will have a ripple effect, travelling outwards like rings of water on a pond after the dramatic splash of a stone. Not only could individual lives and relationships be changed, but the structure of society itself, which is currently suffering from an extremely damaged relationship to the feminine. Both men and women are harmed by a world in which war, violence and exploitation are normalised, and human connection, creativity and our relationship with the natural world are downgraded and sidelined.

Men and women are different. Different does not mean that one is better than the other; it simply means different. It's not possible to write or read a book about life in the female body, or indeed claim that this particular version of human biology is in any way 'special', without acknowledging this difference. In the past, women have felt that in order to compete and win in a man's world, much of what sets us apart must be kept under the radar. This makes a lot of sense when you realise that, historically, our biology has been weaponised against us and used as evidence of our inferiority. All of our powerful biological abilities to create, grow and nurture life have been used to justify our confinement to the domestic sphere, holding us back from all the opportunities in the public sphere that men enjoyed. Any admission of difference, therefore, even in the modern world, brings with it the fear of being discriminated against. However, an awakening is currently taking place in which women are coming to wonder: *Is it me that's inadequate, or is it the world?* We are cyclical beings whose hormones and bodies and brains change and evolve through each monthly cycle and throughout our lifetimes, trying to fit – like square pegs in a round hole – into a world that is built by and for people who don't experience anything like as much variation: men. We have to proudly own our differences, and demand a world that incorporates, accommodates and celebrates them, rather than asking us to pretend they don't exist.

I have called this female cyclical nature the 'matriflux': *matri* comes from the Latin and means not just 'relating to mothers', but also 'relating to women'; *flux* from the Latin 'to flow'. I felt a word was missing to describe this unique experience, the monthly cycle that most of us experience between menarche (our first period) and menopause, but also the wider, ever-shifting nature of being female: the blossoming of puberty; the epic physical changes of pregnancy; the seismic adaptations of motherhood; the mystery of breast milk; the upheaval of perimenopause; the upgrade of menopause, and the final crowning as we become elders. Not all women will experience all of these, but most of us will understand them as part of our physical potential, powers that belong to us as women and to women alone. Some of us will use our energy in other ways, creating projects as well as or instead of babies, and mothering them into life. All of us understand that to be female is a shapeshifting journey that men do not share.

Another word that influenced me to coin the new word 'matriflux', and gave me great pleasure to discover, was 'matrix' – not the 1990s movie cult classic, but a word that today means the epicentre of creation, and which in Middle English meant 'womb'.

I want to be clear that this 'difference' of female biology, this 'matriflux', is not an example of 'biological essentialism'. Male and female people have different physical bodies, this is true, but this does not set any limits on how they are able to live or express themselves. I am a 'biological realist', and I know that, in humans, there are two sexes – male (small motile gametes aka sperm) and female (large gametes aka eggs). Sex is binary and established at conception, male if the sperm carries a Y chromosome, female if it carries an X. The very small number of people with differences of sex development (DSDs, sometimes referred to as 'intersex') are not a 'third sex', but have one of quite a large number of types of DSDs that affect the development of their sex organs in different ways. Most DSDs are male or female specific, and in the extremely rare cases where their anatomies have both male and female features, sex is determined sensitively with the help of medical professionals. Sex in humans is binary and it is different from 'gender' or 'gender identity', the feeling or 'inner sense' that some people (but by no means all) have of whether they are a man or a woman or 'non-binary'. This is not a book about gender identity. It is about the female-sexed body and the cultural, personal, physical and psychological experience of life in such a body. Anyone with a female body may identify as they wish, dress as they wish, be attracted to whomsoever they wish, and be interested in whatever activities or career they wish. We *are* our bodies. And our bodies are tangible and real, and they have a sex, but this does not dictate our life choices or our destiny.

Words are a great source of joy and fascination to me; they are extremely important and powerful, and must be chosen carefully. For the purpose of this book, when I use the word 'woman' I invoke the standard definition of an adult female person, and likewise, when I use the word 'man', I intend it to mean an adult male person. I'm sensitive to the fact that there are people with female bodies who do not wish to see themselves or be defined by others as women, and if you are one such person and are reading this book, I hope that you will understand my decision to keep the language I use rooted in biological reality, and still find the book of value to you. In many ways I'm grateful to the current debates around sex and gender because I think they have forced all of us to reconsider our relationship with our sexed bodies, and, in doing so, to ask what it means to be a 'woman' or a 'mother', and indeed if there is anything special about either of those things. I think that many women are coming to the conclusion that there *is* something special about them, something that they wish to lay claim to or even defend. That is, in part, what this book is about.

As well as the stories we tell about the female body, some of the words we use to tell them also need to change. The area of the vulva is known as the 'pudenda', which comes from the Latin *pudere*, meaning 'to be ashamed'. In Germany, the labia are called the *schamlippen* – the shame lips. Vagina comes from the Latin meaning 'sheath' or 'scabbard', implying that its function is simply a place to put your 'sword'. As someone who has been writing about childbirth for some time, I'm very aware that there is specific terminology here that women have repeatedly asked to be revised but which seems to stubbornly persist. A woman whose labour needs augmenting may have 'failure to progress' written on her notes. If she suffers from a miscarriage, she may be described as having an 'incompetent' or 'insufficient' cervix; if she cannot conceive in the first place, it may be said that she has a 'hostile uterus'. If she wants to have a vaginal birth after a caesarean, this can be called a 'trial of scar'. Many women object to their babies being described as being 'delivered', firstly because it usually implies that someone other than them played a lead role in their newborn's arrival, and secondly because it is also used for pizzas. Women in labour may be infantilised by being called a 'good girl', dehumanised by being described as 'the induction in Room 6' or patronisingly referred to as 'Mum'. Women object to all of this and more, but things nevertheless seem slow to change.

In the process of writing this book I have found example after example of female body parts named after men. Obviously, this is because it was men who 'discovered' them – not just because women, being excluded from science and medicine, were unable to, but also because of the attitude that the female body is a territory that only becomes significant under the male eye. Those little bumps on your nipples? The Montgomery glands, named after Irish obstetrician William Fetherstone Montgomery in 1832. The Fallopian tubes in your uterus? Sixteenth-century Italian anatomist Gabriele Falloppio. Then we have the Skene's glands, located on the vaginal wall, named after Dr Alexander Skene, a nineteenth- century gynaecologist; the Graafian follicles in the ovary, named after Regnier de Graaf in the 1600s, and the Bartholin glands, which secrete lubricating fluid for the vagina during sex, named after Caspar Bartholin the Younger in 1677. Even the G-spot is named after a man: German physician Ernst Gräfenberg – he wrote about it in the early twentieth century and it was posthumously given his initial in the 1980s. The fact that nobody is yet sure whether the 'G-spot' itself actually exists, nor what female ejaculation is or how and why it happens, is symptomatic of the wider problem here: men seem more keen on 'colonising' the female body, naming parts after themselves and sticking their metaphorical flags in them, than in actually understanding their functions, particularly in ways that would be meaningful or helpful to women themselves.

While men have been confidently and unashamedly naming our body parts, we have, through lack of confidence and shame, been unable to name them ourselves. Do you use the word vulva? Do you know the difference between one and your vagina? Where and what is your cervix? Social-media giants like Facebook and Instagram continue to be uncomfortable with words and images relating to women's bodies, censoring posts containing terms such as vagina, menopause, period and clitoris, and removing or covering up pictures that relate to female biology – a situation I've experienced myself many times, even being banned from Facebook in the past for sharing images of natural birth. We still seem to find it difficult to talk about and look at women's bodies in action, and when we teach the next generation of girls about their bodies, we often only do so in relation to their fertility. When I was writing *My Period*, I had to argue the case for including the information that a woman's temperature rises slightly at ovulation, and that, if you're curious, you can track this yourself. The pushback was that this information is only relevant if you're trying to conceive, therefore pre-teen girls didn't need to know it. Hmm. There are an awful lot of things we teach pre-teens that they don't 'need to know' – could there be an underlying anxiety about this specific information because it's awash with female body literacy and also the exact opposite of the approved message for girls in sex ed: 'You can get pregnant at any time of the month.' This isn't true, of course – it's men who are fertile all month long, not women – but we maintain the lie very effectively, partly out of fear that women cannot be trusted to take charge of their own fertility, and partly because it places the onus of unwanted pregnancy solely on the female.

We are still being told myths about the female body, and it's time they were debunked. Women's bodies are not cursed, inadequate, faulty, shameful, hostile, dirty, weak or incompetent. Being female is not a problem to be fixed, or a disease to be cured. Quite the opposite, it is something to take pride in and celebrate. Women are the ultimate source, the creators; from them comes all future life. It's time to reclaim our power.

Chapter 1

Mirror Myths

'The woman wins who calls herself beautiful,
and challenges the world to change to fit her vision.'

NAOMI WOLF, *The Beauty Myth*

I am on an escalator in a leading high-street purveyor of pants and bras in London. As I step off at the top I'm faced with a floor-to-ceiling advertising display for the underwear department: four women inexplicably laughing their heads off as they pose in their smalls. But I pause – something's different. For a moment, I can't quite work it out, and then, the penny slowly drops . . . these women look *real*. Not because one or two of them are older, not because they are not all white and skinny as a hat rack; no, it goes deeper than this. They look real because their skin – the skin of their bodies – is like nothing I've ever seen on a poster before. It's got creases, dimples, saggy bits, moles, spots, stretch marks, lines. I stand and stare for a moment, and I suddenly realise: every single woman I've seen with her body exposed in an advert up until this point in my life has been a fake. I've been repeatedly told that there is a special kind of woman out there with different skin on her body to me, a perfect woman. And I've been lied to.

This doesn't help me twenty minutes later, though, as I huff and puff my way through a dozen different bras, all the time confronted with the bare reality of my naked flesh, reflected from every possible angle in the changing room's mirrored walls. There are a multitude of thoughts I could be having. I could be thinking about the weather, or the design of the bras, or the economics of cryptocurrency. I could even be thinking, as the internet memes instruct me to do, about the wonder of my female form and the three miraculous lives it has produced, each one of them stretching the skin of my abdomen that little bit further, like a celebratory balloon. But I'm not. I'm thinking about each crease, dimple, saggy bit, mole, spot, stretch mark, line, and how much I hate them all. In particular, I'm looking at my stomach; the pregnancy party is long over and it's now a deflated blimp of crinkled latex. I don't want it. I want the fake airbrushed Photoshopped body the adverts made me believe existed. I want the lie back.

I'm not alone in this conundrum – although I'm pretty unusual in that, until three massive babies annihilated my midriff, I used to actually quite like my body. I was slim, with sexy long legs and neat but slightly oversized boobs. I could have any man I liked and, at the time, I believed this signified my overall value, genuinely mistaking the male attention for a positive evaluation of my whole self. What I didn't realise was that if your value is liable to take a nose-dive as soon as your jawline slackens, you're probably better off investing in crypto – now, aged 51, I've spent the past few years readjusting to the new experience of becoming 'invisible' in middle age, and the accompanying realisation that many of the people who used to hang on my every word and tell me I was hilarious and brilliant were doing so because of my outward appearance. They may have said, 'You're so funny/clever/insightful,' but what they actually meant was, 'You're so youthful and conform to practically every beauty standard.' Twenty years ago if I expressed a controversial opinion I was cutting edge or a trailblazer; do the same now and I'm a Karen or a dinosaur – that is, if anybody hears what I'm saying at all.

The Man Inside

This phenomenon of finding that people listen to you and treat you a whole lot better when you are young, female and pert of boob even has a name: 'pretty privilege'. Pretty privilege can, of course, apply to men, too – research has shown that we all have a bias towards more 'attractive' people, meaning that whether you're male or female, good looks can help you in every area,[1] from a quick pay rise to a lighter jail sentence.[2] But there is an added layer of complexity for women, summarised in three words: the male gaze. First coined by the feminist Laura Mulvey in her 1975 essay 'Visual Pleasure and Narrative Cinema', the idea of the 'male gaze' referred originally to the way in which women in film were perceived primarily through the lens of male heterosexual desire.[3] The concept has since widened out to express the way in which the world itself is so often structured around the objectification of women's passive role as one 'to be looked at' and men's active role as 'he who looks'. As females we often live – whether conscious of it or not – in a constant relationship with male approval. Whether this manifests as feeling unable to leave the house without make-up or hit the beach with hairy legs, or, conversely, the decision 'not to bother with any of that stuff' – either way, we very often make these choices under the shadow of the male gaze, which is pervasive and hard to escape.

During puberty, we find ourselves suddenly becoming visible to the male gaze, and may well also begin to be exposed to its dark underbelly: sexual harassment. A culture that objectifies women is permitted to heckle or whistle at them in public – or worse. As we reach perimenopause, we may then find it surprising that the gaze has suddenly averted itself, inciting relief in some and mixed feelings in others at the loss of what can feel like the world's stamp of approval. However we feel or have felt about the gaze, we will almost certainly have internalised it so that it feels like a natural and permanent part of ourselves, and so that the experience of looking in the mirror may often be one of deciding whether or not we approve of our reflection on the patriarchy's behalf. Margaret Atwood put it brilliantly in her novel *The Robber Bride*: 'Even pretending you aren't catering to male fantasies is a male fantasy: pretending you're unseen, pretending you have a life of your own, that you can wash your feet and comb your hair unconscious of the ever-present watcher peering through the keyhole, peering through the keyhole in your own head, if nowhere else. You are a woman with a man inside watching a woman. You are your own voyeur.'[4]

More often than not when we look in the mirror, we allow this 'man inside' to give us the thumbs down, deciding that, rather than meeting the various beauty standards, we will conform instead to the self-loathing that haunts so many females. For women, it is more normal than not normal to dislike or even hate your body, and for this preoccupation to dominate your mind and gnaw away at your self-esteem for a lifetime. Surveys vary, but the percentage of women who don't like what they see in the mirror seems to be somewhere between 60 and 100 per cent. A 2020 survey from the Women and Equalities Committee found that over six out of ten women feel negatively about their bodies,[5] while another from *Glamour* magazine in 2011 produced the shocking statistic that 97 per cent of women have at least one thought along the lines of 'I hate my body' per day, with the average woman telling herself she looks awful thirteen times each day.[6] In recent times, two iconic women have confessed to such habits: Michelle Obama has said there are 'plenty of mornings' when she turns on the bathroom light, takes one look at herself in the mirror, and 'desperately wants to flip it off again', while Emma Thompson has spoken about how she can't just stand still in front of a mirror and look at herself. 'Why would I do that? It's horrifying,' she quipped, before adding, 'Women have been brainwashed all our lives to hate our bodies.'

Now, there is a new way to address our body loathing: GLP-1 receptor agonists popularly known as weight loss jabs: Wegovy, Ozempic, Mounjaro and other leading brands. In the UK, around one in ten people have used these drugs or say they plan to in the near future,[7] and women are around twice as likely to use them as men – experts believe a driving factor for this is likely to be women's long history of social and cultural pressure on their body type, size and weight.[8] Whilst GLP-1 drugs are making a positive difference to many women living with obesity, some feel they are also eating away at what seems to have been a very brief spell of body positivity for larger women. A *Vogue* report in October 2025 found that the fashion industry has done a '360 turn' on plus-sized models, with the widespread use of weight-loss drugs directly implicated for 'normalising thinness'.[9] The pop star Lizzo, who has herself lost weight through conventional methods but who still weighs more than 14 st, has slammed GLP-1 drugs for 'erasing' plus-sized women.[10] In Hollywood, so many A-listers have been dropping in size that the columnist Rose Stokes has labelled 2025 as 'Shrinking Girl Summer', and related trends have begun to spring up, for example the offering of a new cosmetic procedure known as 'Barbie Waist Surgery', in which small incisions are made in the ribs allowing a narrower waist to be remodelled.[11] The long term health effects of the Ozempic trend are not yet known, but concerns are starting to be raised about potential impact on a wide range of areas from mental health to disorders of the optic nerve.[12] Recent research found that those who came off the drugs regained weight four times faster than dieters, and there is growing unease that the cost of the jabs may be transforming obesity, and body image itself, into an issue of wealth and class.[13] Private prescriptions for the drugs currently cost between 100 and 375 pounds a month in the UK, and the global market is expected to be worth 44 billion dollars by 2030.[14] Whilst GLP-1 may be a legitimate help to some, there is no doubt that they have shifted the focus away from body acceptance and back to thinness for women in particular, and that this shift is potentially exploitative of the mirror-based anxiety of all women, particularly those on low-incomes.

> *'That's another thing about being*
> *a certain age that I've noticed:*
> *I try as much as possible not to look in the*
> *mirror. If I pass a mirror, I avert my eyes.'*
>
> NORA EPHRON, *I Feel Bad About My Neck*

Have we always hated our bodies? It's well documented that women's beauty standards have changed over time – a big butt may not have been desirable in the 1990s, but if you wanted to model for seventeenth-century Rubens or emulate a 1950s Marilyn then your curves were something to be celebrated. Waistlines have gone in and out, busts have got bigger and smaller, skin has been pale or tanned, hips ample or svelte, but while the ideal of perfection has continued to shift, women's voices on how they felt if they either met or failed to meet the cultural standard of the day are often missing. Only relatively recently have we had the ability to both be influenced by images of other women on a grand scale, and document extensively our own feelings about our reflections. Women of the past may have been disappointed in their looks – in her poem 'Made When I Was Not Well' the seventeenth-century poet Hester Pulter described her body as a 'loathsome ruined prison . . . spoiled by Time' – and yet they lived before the advent of mass-produced mirrors, fashion photography, movie stars, social media and the concept of 'cosmetic surgery'.[15] These ingredients seem to be providing twenty-first-century women with the perfect storm: impossible standards, inevitable self-loathing and the tantalising promise of a solution.

Barbie Girls

There is not a single body part that some woman, somewhere, will not say she hates about herself. Correspondingly, there is not a single body part that a surgeon, somewhere, will not offer to transform for you. Originally developed for wounded soldiers and people with injuries, burns and disfigurements, cosmetic surgery is now a booming global business, currently worth over 70 billion dollars,[16] and expected to be worth 205 billion dollars globally by 2030.[17] Parts of our bodies that don't seem to conform – the sagging belly, the too-small breasts, even the unruly vulva – can now be brought into line for the cost of a second-hand motor – around £6,000 for your tummy tuck[18]; £7,000 for your boob job[19]; and labiaplasty, a (ahem) snip at around £4,000.[20]

If you've not heard of labiaplasty, it's surgery on the labia – the inner and outer 'lips' of the vulva – a trimming of the folds of skin that surround the vaginal opening. Although sometimes performed to meet a clinical need, labiaplasty is usually done for entirely cosmetic reasons. Worldwide, the number of labiaplasty procedures carried out in 2023 reached just over 189,000,[21] an increase of 42.2 per cent compared to 2018 and up 99 per cent compared to 2015. Researchers believe the ever-increasing demand is largely due to rising exposure to pornography, in which the vulva is often presented as hairless and 'neat', and doctors report that women who seek labiaplasty will often show pictures of Photoshopped or pornified labia and ask to be made to look similarly 'tidy' and 'normal'.[22] 'Generally speaking, a labiaplasty does to your vertical lips what a barber does to your split ends,' states the website Healthline.[23] One doctor in Laguna Beach, California, has invented a version of labiaplasty known as 'The Barbie', in which the labia minora are completely removed, resulting in a 'clamshell aesthetic',[24] which his website claims will 'restore femininity'.[25] The definition of 'femininity' has changed and shifted over the decades, but right now, in 2026, it's 'hyper' – a plastic and pornified version of womanhood that invites us to present ourselves as identikit dolls all the way from our snatched and sculpted faces to our hairless and unreal vulvas. Some suggest this overall aesthetic, dubbed 'bimbocore' or 'bimbofem' in the early 2020s, is a feminist reclamation of confident, empowered femininity – but is it really empowering to erase all trace of individuality, and if so, why aren't men doing it?

In spite of initiatives to inform teenage girls that vulvas come in an infinite variety of shapes and sizes, and that all are normal, the number of women of all ages requesting surgery to make their bodies conform to a homogenised ideal continues to rise.[26] Labia that are not 'neat' or 'tidy' have, of course, become much more obvious to women in recent years, due to another current trend with its roots in pornography – the complete removal of pubic hair. Women throughout history have always trimmed and depilated, and there does seem to be a long-standing relationship between innocence and hairlessness versus untamed pubes and wild sexuality. Ironic, then, that the current fashion of totally bald nethers seems to have some connection to porn, in which both male and female actors often remove all hair to expose and emphasise the genitals for the cameras. Add to this another porn-inspired trend: 'bleaching', using lasers or creams to make the skin around the anus or vulva appear lighter and therefore more like the rest of the skin on the body, and the aspirational female vulva, rather than being wild and untamed, certainly does seem a lot like the hairless, slitless, smooth and indifferent plastic Barbie dolls'. You can even go further and make sure it doesn't actually smell like a vulva either – a vast selection of completely unnecessary products and so-called 'intimate washes' (by which they mean, but would of course never say, vulva soap) capitalise on women's insecurities in a global market currently worth over 3 billion dollars. Literally nobody needs vulva soap: the vagina (the part *inside*) is self-cleaning and the vulva (the part *outside*) can be washed with water and, if necessary, any mild soap. Some of these attempts to be 'fresh' can even be dangerous: in 2018 a Missouri jury awarded over 4 billion dollars to twenty-two women who claimed that their ovarian cancer was caused by using Johnson & Johnson talc.[27] There is no equivalent industry that plays on the insecurities of men.

Do we just not want to be 'real' any more? There is perhaps something more passive about the doll vulva than the messy, bloody, smelly, hairy, technicolour 'real' one. Stripped of every possible sign of our animal nature, our reproductive capacity and our living, breathing mortality, the doll vulva presents itself only as a series of expectant orifices without much of a story to tell. The pressure on teenage girls and younger women to make a choice between two polar extremes – groomed to the point of every trace of reality being hidden, or sensual and wild in a way that mainstream culture seems to disapprove of – may be unprecedented in the way it is currently manifesting in body modification and surgery but nevertheless feels familiar in its reflection of the age-old tropes of virgin and whore. The 'real' woman – sensual, sexual, life-creating – has a power that has cast fear into men for millennia, and women have long had to adapt themselves, tone themselves down, make themselves smaller and compromise on their 'realness', in an attempt to make life easier under the male gaze. At a time when there is increased focus on the notion of being 'gender non-conforming', it seems as if the female body has never been under more pressure to conform, caught between two polar extremes of hyperfemininity at one end, and total rejection of the female body at the other through non-binary or trans identities, with the breasts flattened by binders or surgically removed through so-called 'gender-affirming surgery'. At both extremes of the spectrum the female body must change dramatically in order to be accepted.

At menarche, this aspect of being female often becomes apparent to a young girl for the first time, with the revelation that her body is rapidly changing into a being that will henceforth not only be objectified, but also potentially judged to be unwanted or even repulsive lest she work hard to modify it. The pubic hair that is appearing must never be seen. Should it be removed? And what about the period blood? Might that leak out and cause humiliation in the school corridor? And the breasts? Men are noticing them, approving of them. Approval is a good thing, right? So then why does it feel so uncomfortable? Why does it feel as if, suddenly, so many aspects of the body should be kept hidden? What was once a vehicle for tree-climbing, cartwheeling, running and jumping for joy has evolved overnight into something more akin to an unexploded bomb. For some, this newfound complexity can result in mental ill health such as self-harm, anorexia or bulimia, all of which are three times more likely in young girls than in young boys.[28] The causes of eating disorders are complex and not fully understood, and may differ from person to person, with genetic, environmental, social and psychological components. The journalist Hadley Freeman, who was hospitalised for three years as a teenager with anorexia and has now written a book about it, *Good Girls*, feels that the idea that teenage girls develop anorexia because they are 'silly women wanting to look like models' is sexist and 'condescending'.[29] Instead, she describes how, for her, the illness represented a 'fear of womanhood'. 'The things that led up to it for me are not what everyone always says – it has nothing to do with fashion models and magazine and celebrities . . . this is the truth about anorexia, it's a fear of womanhood,' she told journalist Julie Bindel. 'This is something that no one ever seems to understand. Anorexia comes on in adolescence, invariably, always, and it's, I think, girls who have a fear of becoming women because of either their fear of being sexualised, their fear of leaving their mother, their fear of becoming their mother, their fear of what being a woman means, a desire to stay a child.'[30]

This 'fear of womanhood' that Freeman describes has manifested in a new way in the past decade, with a sudden explosion in numbers of adolescent girls with gender dysphoria. Defined by the NHS as a 'sense of unease a person may have because of a mismatch between their biological sex and gender identity', gender dysphoria is most often expressed as a desire to identify as non-binary (neither male nor female) or transgender.[31]

In 2009 in England, there were thirty-two girls and forty boys referred to the Gender Identity Development Service (GIDS) at London's Tavistock and Portman NHS Foundation Trust. In 2021 there were almost 5,000, twice the number of referrals in the previous year. And of that 5,000, the largest group – about two-thirds – were adolescent girls.[32] These figures are yet to be fully understood. The current rise in acceptance for different ways of identifying cannot explain why so many teenage girls – rather than any other demographic – are wishing to be boys instead, and, as a result, 'binding' and hoping to one day have 'top surgery' (elective mastectomy), asking to be referred to as 'he', requesting medication to 'block' puberty, and taking testosterone, the latter of which can cause irreversible changes such as a deepened voice and facial hair growth. As the organisation Transgender Trend put it in evidence they submitted to the UK Parliament, 'There is no understanding nor any explanation or hypothesis as to why "increased trans visibility" has influenced predominantly teenage girls, particularly when the trans people who are more visible are largely middle-aged males, often portraying the glamorised version of womanhood young girls are rejecting.'[33]

Vulva Power

The female body is at its most confronting when it is in action. I've experienced this first hand when I've been banned from social media for sharing images of childbirth – most memorably once on the same day that Kim Kardashian's oily and airbrushed bum on the cover of *PAPER* magazine was said to be 'breaking the internet'. Taking to Twitter, I shared a picture of Kim's internet-breaking bottom, and the birthing bottom, side by side, and asked, 'How come some bums are OK and some bums are not?' But I already knew the answer. A woman's birthing bottom is real and active and powerful and not remotely concerned with how it looks; Kardashian's rump was the opposite – fake, passive and entirely in service of the male gaze. It's this confrontation with a new, almost secret and hidden aspect of our female bodies that leads some women to find childbirth transformative. When the visionary eco-feminist artist Monica Sjöö gave birth to her second baby at home in the late 1960s, it changed the entire direction of her creativity. 'I found that birth so extraordinary and very much a spiritual/physical almost religious experience. I could find NO split between the mind/body that we are supposed to believe in – and I couldn't understand that we women can be called "weak" when our beings are capable of such strength as creation through birth,' she said.[34] Shortly after that, in 1968, Sjöö painted her iconic 'God Giving Birth', which depicts a Black woman giving birth to the universe. The power of the picture, which shows the woman, upright, with a baby's head emerging from her vulva, was clear: it was removed from two different exhibitions and Sjöö was threatened with prosecution for blasphemy and obscenity. A print of it now hangs on my upstairs landing – but would I dare display it in my kitchen? Where it is, only my eye-rolling teenagers and the occasional house guest are exposed to its powerful message. Maybe that's enough.

The vulva – in particular when it is raw, active, and not being displayed purely in the service of men – has the power to shock unlike arguably any other body part, male or female. Carved images of women proudly displaying their vulvas, known as 'sheela na gigs', can be found on churches and other buildings in Western Europe. We don't really know the exact reason for sheela na gigs, although they are often placed over doorways, leading some to speculate that they represent the female as the universal gateway of life. Many of them were placed high up, out of sight, perhaps because they were a taboo throwback to paganism, or perhaps because they were something secret and powerful, a talisman of life and death. They are often beloved of midwives, most notably Ina May Gaskin, who believes the icons, with their vulvas held open wide, were intended to 'reassure young women about the capabilities of their bodies in birth . . . the vulva of the crouching figure is open enough to accommodate her own head. Such a sight is quite encouraging to a woman in labor,' as she writes in her bestselling *Guide to Childbirth*. Whatever their purpose, sheela na gigs have upset people through the ages, from horrified Victorian clergy, to vandals as recently as 2004 who destroyed one in West Sussex,[35] to the Catholic Church in 1631, which instructed its parish priests in Tuam to destroy these 'gross images with unpleasant aspects'.[36] In the first half of the twentieth century, a 'mother and baby' home operated in Tuam, a Catholic-run institution for unmarried mothers where it was later discovered that 796 infants had died and been buried in unmarked graves. Whilst three hundred years passed between these two events, they are nevertheless connected by a dangerous anger towards female sexuality and women's life-giving power.

There is some evidence that, in the further reaches of history, we have not always felt this way. Stone Age sites have many examples of carved 'V' shapes, triangles and more obvious vulvas,[37] suggesting that this part of the body was seen as the true source of power in the world, and the feminine was worshipped. Early Christianity retained some of this legacy, with sheela na gigs, and also persistent vulvic shapes in medieval manuscripts,[38] in which the wounds of Christ – along with their life-giving power – are portrayed as very vulva-like, in a classic almond shape known as the mandorla (think of the shape that is made when two equally sized circles overlap, also known as the '*vesica piscis*').[39] In researching this, I had a sudden flashback to my Catholic primary school, where girls would have 'medals of Our Lady' – a depiction of Mary and often the same 'almond-shaped' mandorla. And, of course, Our Lady herself is just another iteration of the Divine Feminine with some pointing out that her depictions in her flowing robes do look a bit . . . er . . . vulva like, and some imagery, such as Our Lady of Guadalupe in Mexico, looking almost more yonic than human. Other times Mary is shown with her robes making a triangular shape – for example, in some South American icons such as Our Lady of the Rosary in

Guatemala – each side of the triangle perhaps representing the trinity of womanhood (maiden, mother and crone) or perhaps a connection to the 'V' or triangle we see as far back as the Stone Age as a symbol of the pubic area, the uterus and the feminine.[40] Each culture has its goddesses or representations of female power, and some remain: the Hindu goddess Kali, for example, is a ferocious symbol of power – complex, destructive, unapologetic and wild. Under the layers of shame and objectification with which most modern women are familiar, the vulva tells a very different story.

> 'La mar es posa bona si veu el cony d'una dona.'
> *'The sea calms down if it sees a woman's cunt.'*
>
> CATALAN SAYING

If you've never thought about your vagina and vulva as remotely powerful, you might be surprised to learn of 'anasyrma', otherwise known as 'raising the skirt'. This gesture, of lifting up your clothing to expose your vulva, is as old as humanity, and 'can be found in the history, folklore, or mythology of every country or culture', as Catherine Blackledge explains in her book *Raising the Skirt: The Unsung Power of the Vagina*. 'Vaginas, the raising the skirt stories all say, are so powerful that if a woman lifts her skirt to reveal her genitalia, she can make a vast array of extraordinary actions happen. Displaying the vagina in this way gives women the power to control the elements: calming the sea to protect sea-faring spouses, subduing storms . . . Raising the skirt is also an apotropaic act – capable of averting evil: vaginal display scares away attacking bears or lions, exorcises demons and drives out the devil.'[41]

There are multiple examples of anasyrma in Blackledge's book, from the Kom people of West Cameroon who practise 'Anlu', a ritual display of the vulva as a way of symbolically disciplining men who have committed offences against them; to the myth of Baubo, who flashed her vagina to make Demeter laugh and is said to have inspired her own cult featuring 'face in body' statues with, you guessed it, visible vulvas; to multiple tales of women stopping war or avenging violence with this powerful statement of 'Enough'. Each story from a wide range of cultures and situations seems to have the same common denominator – a vulva can stop you in your tracks and make you reconsider in a way that words, money or even a gun cannot. Grand speeches, bribes or threats of violence do not seem to have the same quiet, very slightly humorous power as this female body part. Very much more recently, we saw anasyrma in action in the Scottish Parliament, when protester Elaine Miller raised her skirt in the public gallery. Miller, who was protesting against the Gender Recognition Reform Bill, and in particular the issue of convicted male rapists being housed in the female estate, did not actually expose her vulva but instead wore thick flesh-coloured tights with a large triangle of fake fur attached. 'Women lifting their skirt is an ancient and global protest,' she told me. 'I decided that if my government were going to remove my sex-based rights then I would shock them with the power of my sex. It certainly caught the attention of my elected representatives, and I'd say it was a successful political protest. I have no regrets.' The reaction to Elaine's gesture confirms the enduring power of anasyrma: she was described as a 'sex offender' and a police investigation was launched – concluding, somewhat predictably, that no offence had been committed.[42]

The vulva could be seen as the absolute emblem of our femaleness, and a microcosm of the shame and stigma that surrounds the female form and which is at the root of many women's lack of confidence and pride in their entire body. It's therefore an area to potentially focus on if you are interested in changing how you feel when you look in the mirror. The idea of publicly exposing your vulva – real or fake – may be a bridge too far, but women are reclaiming this part of their body in other slightly less dramatic ways. For some, this may simply be the radical act of looking at your vulva in a mirror. First suggested (in print at least) in the seminal book *Our Bodies, Ourselves*, published in 1970 and now considered a feminist turning point, even this seemingly straightforward activity is unnerving to some, in spite of the fact that as well as potentially being empowering, it could also help you to get a better idea of what's 'normal' for you, and therefore keep an eye out for any changes and possible health issues. Looking at yourself like this is rebellion, a way of taking ownership of this body part which for many women is most often seen not by them, but by their sexual partners or their doctors. 'We emphasize that you take a mirror and examine yourself. Touch yourself, smell yourself, even taste your own secretions,' said the original edition of *Our Bodies, Ourselves*. 'After all, you are your body and you are not obscene.'[43]

Five decades later, the option exists to make a 'vulva positive' statement, with vulva jewellery, art or clothing in a vulva print – most recently worn by actress Gillian Anderson at the 2024 Golden Globes (although she erroneously told reporters her frock was embroidered with 'vaginas' – the mix-up between these two body parts just isn't going away in a hurry).[44] Those feeling a little bolder can have a portrait of their vulva painted or photographed, or even a cast made to display on their wall. Danielle Reader is a photographer from Somerset who creates portraits of women naked in nature, and had her own vulva – and breasts, too – cast by a professional in 2022. 'I follow a lot of body-positive accounts on Instagram because of my own photography work, so that's how I got the idea,' she told me. 'I think I've always appreciated the female form and love any artistic takes on it. I originally booked to just get my breasts done, and then I think I had a "f*** it" moment and thought, *I'll get my vulva done at the same time!*' Both casts are now proudly displayed on the wall of her house, says Danielle, and she hopes it will be empowering, not just for her, but also for her young daughter. 'I also want to normalise the female form for her and for her to know that there should be no shame surrounding her body. She is able to confidently and correctly name body parts, which I don't think is something I could have done when I was younger!'

This body literacy that Danielle is giving her daughter could potentially be a life-changing, or even life-saving, gift, but will nevertheless set her apart as unusual. A 2019 survey found that 73 per cent of women were confused as to what a vulva was. Another survey, conducted by UK health professionals in 2021, showed that only 9 per cent of Britons could label all parts of the vulva, 37 per cent mislabelled the clitoris, and less than half (46 per cent) knew that women have three holes.[45] The widespread shame and disrespect for the female body continues to manifest in this potentially dangerous lack of knowledge, which charities like the Eve Appeal work hard to address with cancer prevention campaigns such as #KnowYourBody. 'Gynae cancers deserve more air time, the symptoms are too little known, and we still need to smash shame, taboos and embarrassment about all things gynae,' their website states. 'Knowing your body means knowing what your reproductive organs are called and what the signs and symptoms of gynae cancers are, so that you can look out for them and seek medical advice if needed.'[46]

Life-threatening illnesses aside, it can be harder to love a body that causes you regular discomfort, pain or even agony, and yet this is common for women, whether it be debilitating period cramps, or pain from underlying conditions that their periods take the blame for. The gap in healthcare professionals' understanding of the female body, and the real-life impact this has on us each and every day – for example, the eight years it can take from first symptom to diagnosis of endometriosis – is becoming well documented.[47] Many women now know some of the shocking statistics around the 'gender health gap'; for example, that women's bodies were not included in clinical trials until 1993, or that women presenting with health issues are often 'gaslit' by professionals into thinking it's all in their head – a throwback to the concept of 'hysteria'. Hysteria – this idea from the Ancient Greeks that the uterus can literally break free and travel around the body, causing blockages, pain and chaos, seems like the perfect metaphor for the extreme discomfort the patriarchy feels about women who refuse to be managed, contained and controlled. Nevertheless, the idea has persisted throughout the centuries, evolving slowly over time to encompass and explain away almost every problem a woman may present with, from unhappiness in her marriage, to a horrible sex life, to infertility, to pain, to depression, to psychosis – all of it caused simply by the condition of being female itself. Like a giant, patriarchal shrug, this 'woman blaming' is convenient, effectively meaning that nothing can be done and nothing needs to change. And while we may feel that such attitudes belong in the history books, women continue to report both a lack of awareness from doctors of typically female health issues, and a consistent pattern of not being taken seriously and being 'fobbed off'.[48] Just as we find the reality of the female body confronting, so, too, it seems, do we find it equally hard to truly listen to women's voices.

The Penis Is the Male Clitoris

> *'What's the difference between the clitoris and a pub? Every man knows how to find a pub.'*

While our pain has never been taken seriously, neither has our pleasure. Our world may be dominated by the male gaze, and we may be bombarded by hypersexualised images of women, but the lack of actual knowledge about female sexual anatomy and function makes for a stark contrast. Even now, more than two decades into the twenty-first century, both schoolteachers and parents are somewhat nervous about telling young girls about this long-misunderstood and overlooked part of their bodies – the clitoris, which still gets little or no attention in biology or sex ed. When it is mentioned at all, the clitoris is often referred to as 'pea-sized', whereas we now know that this is vastly inaccurate and does women a huge disservice. And like books and resources for young people on sex ed, anatomy books for trainee health professionals have also had very little to say about the clitoris. 'When I was studying to be a surgeon, the textbook we used had a lot to say about the penis – four pages – but the clitoris was almost completely omitted,' says Australian urologist Professor Helen O'Connell.[49] It's O'Connell whom we have to thank for our current understanding of the clitoris – it was she who published the first extensive anatomical study in 1998, and subsequently mapped it further using MRI in 2005. You may perhaps be familiar with the three-dimensional shape the MRI revealed – not a 'pea' at all, but a large internal structure, resembling a wishbone. Only 10 per cent of the clitoris is visible, the rest is hidden, surrounding the vaginal opening, filled with more than 10,000 nerve fibres, and extending to around 9 cm when aroused.[50]

From the start of her career, O'Connell, who says she was 'raised a little bit rebelliously', noticed the framing of the female body as a lesser version of the male, everywhere she looked.[51] In her textbooks she found phrases like 'failure', 'lacking' and 'poorly developed' in descriptions of the female anatomy, describing these body parts consistently for their comparative faults and weaknesses to the male default. O'Connell noted, too, the history of doctors, most notably the Victorian Isaac Baker Brown, in removing the clitoris surgically to cure diseases, such as epilepsy and, of course, 'hysteria'. In the early Nineties, O'Connell noticed the great care paid to preserving the sexual function of males undergoing prostate surgery, but could find no corresponding studies into clitoral nerves and sensation. Whether by the surgeon's knife or the textbook writer's pen, the clitoris has been, and continues to be, dismissed, sidelined and removed as unimportant.

The roots of our anatomical oversights and confusions can be traced deep: all the way back to good old Aristotle (who else?!). It's quite incredible, really, when you consider how an idea – in Aristotle's case, 'women are deformed men' – can be put forward, and then form the basis for millennia of thought and research, becoming an eternal human blind spot that only out-of-the-box thinkers like Helen O'Connell can upturn. After Aristotle came other Greek physicians, most of whom decided that something was going 'wrong' in the development of female babies that meant the penis couldn't 'unfurl' and instead stayed on the inside. When Renaissance anatomists actually began to dissect female cadavers, they superimposed their existing bias onto their findings, creating drawings that confirmed the vagina was an 'interior penis', in spite of the evidence to the contrary that was right in front of their eyes. And even today this bias persists in the stories we tell about male and female bodies; for example, you sometimes hear that all foetuses begin life as female but *develop further* into males with the presence of the Y chromosome. This is not really the case: sex is determined at conception, depending on whether the sperm is carrying an X or a Y chromosome. From this male-dominated narrative, however, we arrive at the idea that the female is a sort of 'underdeveloped male' and that therefore the clitoris is the female penis. This version of reality somehow feels more acceptable than the alternative perspective that the penis is the male clitoris.

As females, our capacity for pleasure is unlimited in a way that males may envy: arguably we are built for orgasmic pleasure in a way that they are simply not. A woman may have as many orgasms in a day as she has time and inclination for, while a man has limits. In spite of this incredible female capacity, overall, men seem to be having the most orgasms. Like all areas of women's bodies, there is a huge lack of research into our pleasure, particularly in comparison to men's. What we do know, however, consistently highlights a so-called 'orgasm gap' – which applies particularly to heterosexual couples. One large study in the US in 2017 found that the demographic most likely to orgasm during sex were heterosexual men (95 per cent), while the group least likely to orgasm were heterosexual women (65 per cent) – the lowest of all groups studied.[52] Knowledge of the female body makes a difference: several studies have found that lesbian couples are having more orgasms, and other studies suggest that female nurses and doctors, with their extra anatomical awareness, are more likely to have multiple orgasms.[53] Articles on this topic are often careful to reiterate that men are not to blame for this, and yet we do know that women have more orgasms masturbating alone than they do when having sex with a partner – 39 per cent versus 6 per cent, according to one study,[54] and a 2021 survey found that these solo orgasms were better, too.[55] According to researchers, we also have a culturally baked-in belief that men are more entitled to orgasm than women; several different studies at the University of Michigan in 2021 found that, when it came to perceptions of heterosexual couples, as many as three-quarters of people agreed that male climax was of greater importance than female.[56]

Take Up Space

Our bias against the female body has both deep roots and long tendrils, reaching into every area of women's lives and slowly but surely twisting its way around anything and everything, from whether we struggle to stand naked in front of the mirror, to a potential lifetime of missed orgasms. There's even a link between these two[57]: women who feel confident in their body image have better sex with more orgasms.[58] There's research to prove this, not that we need it, because I bet there's not a single woman reading this who hasn't, at some point, had her sexual or romantic life impacted by how she feels about the way she looks – perhaps her weight, perhaps her ageing process, maybe a comment about her naked body that a partner has made that has stuck in her mind. The messaging that our female bodies are in some way lacking is often accompanied with a side order of 'you can't win' – always we must tread a fine line between too much and too little. We can be too lusty, too loud, too opinionated, too fat, too hairy, too confident and probably too orgasmic. But careful: hold back and we may find we are too quiet, too boring, too thin or too frigid. As mothers we slam even harder between this rock and hard place: we are too attached, too involved, too smothering, too obsessed with our kids, we have let ourselves go, we are frumpy or matronly. But careful: if we keep our old selves alive too enthusiastically we may be too distant, too self-obsessed, too career focused, too ambitious. We must work like we don't have kids and mother like we don't work. For all our lives as women we harbour desires to be complex, multifaceted, nuanced, vibrant, real and fully human, yet so often we can find ourselves butting up against the bars of a cage that keeps us from this rich and complete life.

In the 1990s, I joined a gym – probably, whether I realised it or not, under the influence of Princess Diana, who was so often papped leaving one in her shorts and sunglasses. It's the only explanation I can think of for why I decided I needed to work out four times a week, aged 20, my body brand new and flawless. At my first couple of sessions, I was given a plan by an instructor, who told me that on each visit I should circulate the various machines, and on each one always use only the very lowest weights for a high number of reps. 'NEVER', they told me (and yes, they were male), 'NEVER use heavy weights. If you lift heavy weights, you'll get big.' It was taken as an absolute given that 'getting big' was a horror I would never wish to experience, and I dutifully obeyed, not thinking to question the reasoning, or why indeed there was a whole section of the gym – the one with barbells and mirrors – that it was assumed I would never wish to enter. I went round in circles, obediently lifting my low weights on high reps for a year or so, and then quit, my body as young and flexible – and 'small' – as it had been when I joined. Being 'small' or 'getting smaller' is a lifetime body goal for many women – in her seminal book *The Beauty Myth* Naomi Wolf called this the 'One Stone Solution', the idea that losing 14 lbs is the only thing that stands between us and the happiness that would come from being our ideal selves. The message that our lives would improve if only there were less of us, if only we made our bodies as small and as negligible as possible – now being repeated in its latest iteration of GLP-1 weight-loss drugs – is a powerful one.

Twenty-five years after my first gym membership, three children and a pandemic later, I decided – this time more out of self-love and care than vanity – that I needed to do something about my health and fitness. My memory flashed back to the instructor's advice, and although now things in the gym seemed a little more laid-back – 'Do what you like!' – there was still an invisible line of division between the area with the machines and treadmills (mixed sex) and the area with the free weights and benches (male only). Was this a new glass ceiling that, in spite of a lifetime of feminism, I'd only just noticed? This time, in my fuck-it-forties rather than my toe-the-line-twenties, I stared at the free weights area and wondered, *What if I went in?* And, *What if I 'got big'*? Why had the man in my Nineties gym told me what I didn't want? And why the heck had I let him?! To begin with, I still didn't cross the line. *How would a middle-aged, out-of-shape woman fatally trapped under a barbell be dealt with by a small group of muscle-bound 25-year-olds?* was my main concern. Also,

I wasn't quite sure what I was doing, and while that didn't particularly bother me, I knew it would lay me wide open, not so much to humilitation, but – much worse by far – to mansplaining. I watched from a distance, and bided my time.

With the idea of lifting weights still calling to me, I stumbled by accident into a class called Body Pump, which, if you haven't tried it yourself, consists of 'squats, deadlifts, clean and presses, lunges, bicep curls, push-ups, chest presses, overhead presses and crunches'. Before I knew it, I was lifting a barbell repeatedly over my head, and loving it. I could lift 5 kg, maybe even 7.5 kg. I felt strong. But another woman who came to the same class kept catching my attention. She was younger than me, perhaps in her thirties, and quite beautiful. She was lifting massive weights, which made my 5 kg look like pick-and-mix sweets. And she was big. Really big – her muscles were huge. But the thing that suddenly struck me as I watched her lift one day was that, perhaps for the first time in my life, I was looking at another woman and instead of thinking, *I wish I was thin like her*, I was thinking something different: *I wish I was strong like her.*

The journey towards getting strong is still in progress for me, but it's challenged my thinking about my own body and the female body itself. I'm not alone: the trend for women's weightlifting has been rising steadily since it debuted at the Olympics in 2000, with many now realising the benefits for self-esteem,[59] mental health,[60] bone density (and the prevention of osteoperosis),[61] increased metabolism (pass the cheese), improved cardiovascular health,[62] and even reduced mortality.[63] For women in the cloudy area of 'perimenopause', strength training is considered to be particularly beneficial, for all the reasons already listed, and because midlife is a time when women tend to gain fat and lose muscle mass. Personally, though, more than any of these reasons, I like it because it feels disobedient, counter-cultural, even *feminist* to get strong and maybe even, one day, get big. It feels like something the women in my 'red thread' – my mother, her mother, her mother's mother, and even my 20-year-old self – would have been discouraged from doing. For this reason alone, I want to experience it. I want to lift those weights over my head for the women who couldn't, or who still can't.

And in some ways, although strength training is new to me, it feels familiar, because it feels like childbirth, and it feels like motherhood. I've already pushed my body to its absolute limits, and gone through the pain barrier, and kept going when every shred of me wanted to quit. I've already felt the raw power of my body, and the accomplishment of extreme endurance. And, through three pregnancies, I've already 'got big'. Unimaginably big. If the cultural demand of femininity is in some part about being as 'small' as possible, dieting with the sole focus of weighing less, exercising but making sure we don't build muscle, apologising before we quietly speak, sitting with our legs together rather than 'manspreading' and working in the same roles for less money or less acclaim, then the reality of the female body is extremely disruptive to all this. Everything about it is underestimated: the clitoris is a pea; the vagina may be too narrow; the breasts may not make enough milk. We are told not just that we *must* be small, but that we *are* small. The female body says, 'No.' It says, 'Watch me bleed without dying; watch me shapeshift, right before your eyes; watch me have multiple orgasms; see my almost effortless power and strength as I grow bigger than you think is possible, then watch me show the courage of a warrior while my body opens up wider than wide.' Our culture tells us one story about the female sex and our bodies tell a completely different one, loudly. And, each month, we receive a vivid red reminder of this power, which the world tells us repeatedly to keep hidden away.

Chapter 2
Blood Myths

'Women are tired of the ways men bleed.'

JUDY GRAHN

Carved into the limestone wall of a cave in the Dordogne, the Venus of Laussel lay hidden for 20,000 years. I like to imagine her there, solid and unchanging all that time, holding tight to her secrets as the world outside spins chaotically through each millennium. Forty-six centimetres high, she is a woman with expansive curves: voluptuous breasts, wide hips and thighs, and a rounded, protruding belly. Faceless, her hair drapes onto her left shoulder, and her contours still bear the traces of a time when they were painted red with ochre. Her left hand rests over her womb, and in her right she holds a horn, distinctly marked with thirteen notches.

Why thirteen? This number might make you immediately think of Friday the thirteenth, or perhaps you know that Judas was said to be the thirteenth guest at the Last Supper, or that there are thirteen witches in a coven, thirteen knots in a noose, and thirteen steps to the gallows. In the Norse myth, Loki attends a dinner party in Valhalla and tricks the blind god Hodr into killing Baldr, god of light and goodness. And, just like Judas Iscariot, Loki was also the thirteenth guest. But there's another, hidden story to the number thirteen. Because before anyone had heard the stories of Judas or Loki, thirteen was said to be associated with the moon, with the menstrual cycle, and with the sacred feminine. The passage of a year, in a time before the calendar we know now, would have been marked by thirteen moons. Similarly, a year would contain thirteen menstrual cycles. And the thirteenth day of each of those cycles would mark the peak – the time of ovulation, and maximum fertility – just as it could also represent the countdown of days from ovulation to the next period.

Friday, bound together in our consciousness with thirteen, also has a hidden story. It's the only day of the week to be named after a female – the proto-Germanic goddess Frija (who is thought to have evolved into two other Norse goddesses: Freya and Frigg).[1] Frija, Freya and Frigg are all *völvas,* Viking practitioners of Norse magic known as *seidr.*[2] *Völvas* were shamans, who travelled alone from place to place, using ceremony to divine the future and intervene in the course of fate. They carried a large staff, thought to be the origin of the magic wand, and they were exclusively female. When Norse tribes converted to Christianity, it is said that Freya was labelled a witch and banished to the mountains, where each Friday she would convene a group of eleven other witches and the devil to plot disasters for the coming week. So both Friday and the number thirteen represent the female and the divine feminine, upon which the patriarchal forces of early Christianity were extremely determined to put a negative spin. Superstition leads to fear; anxiety about the potential female power to make 'bad things happen', urges people to mistrust the feminine, even if they are female themselves.

The Venus of Laussel points to her womb and holds the number thirteen aloft. Although she is faceless, she nevertheless seems to confidently meet our gaze and say, 'This is my superpower.' Perhaps she has the confidence of a woman from a time in which the female, the cycles and menstrual blood itself were all respected and venerated as the life source. Times have changed. Although the associations between thirteen and the moon and female cycles have now mostly been forgotten, the number is still mistrusted and considered a 'rogue' number – where twelve is often held to be symbolic of order and perfection, thirteen can be thought of as awkward, indivisible and, frankly, odd. You might even go so far as to say that the neat and predictable twelve is the 'male' to the wild, untameable and somewhat more 'female' thirteen.

The idea that the female body – as well as a woman's thoughts, emotions and behaviours – is messy, erratic, defective and in need of control or management is rampant. It pervades throughout history and across cultures, and menstruation appears to be a crucible for this phenomenon like no other. As mentioned in Chapter 1, Aristotle – widely known as the biggest misogynist of antiquity – wrote that 'the female is, as it were, a deformed male', and he seemed to be particularly confused about periods, poor chap. He believed that menstrual blood was the female equivalent of male semen, but that, unlike semen, it was 'impure' because it lacked the magical ingredient of 'soul'. It was only men, with their superior biology, therefore, who brought anything to the table during conception, depositing the miraculous gift of human spirit into women's wombs, where the soulless menstrual blood would merely provide the basics.

For Aristotle, this explained why periods stop during pregnancy. For the rest of us, it demonstrates quite nicely the origins of sexist ideas that still persist today – that women's bodies, far from being the ultimate life source, are merely containers or vessels for man's creation, and that we are lesser than men simply by nature of our biology. Or, as Aristotle put it, 'The female is a female by virtue of a certain lack of qualities – a natural defectiveness.' This 'defectiveness' became the widely used justification for women being held back from education and public life and instead confined to the home, our menstruation a visible symbol of both our sole purpose – reproduction – and our inadequacy. But wherever there is a negative story about women and their bodies, *look again*. Because it is always here that you will find, hidden away just like the Venus of Laussel herself, a different story: the truth of female power.

Bad Blood

'Never trust a creature that bleeds for five days and doesn't die.'

South Park

There seems to be a pervading fear of menstrual blood itself that shows up everywhere from popular culture to Pliny – another bloke from antiquity, this time Rome – who wrote that:

> *Contact with it turns new wine sour, crops touched by it become barren . . . seed in gardens are dried up, the fruit of trees falls off, the edge of steel and the gleam of ivory are dulled, hives of bees die, even bronze and iron are at once seized by rust, and a horrible smell fills the air; to taste it drives dogs mad and infects their bites with an incurable poison.*

Pliny lived around 2,000 years ago, but as recently as a hundred years ago some people believed that the proximity of a menstruating woman could stop bread from rising, jam from setting or milk turning to butter. So powerful was a woman on her period, apparently, that even her breath could cause plants to wilt, and she could kill insects that infect crops just by walking through a field (which, to be fair, actually sounds quite useful). These ideas may sound like superstition or folklore, but in fact, they had real scientific support. In the 1920s, the Hungarian-born American paediatrician Béla Schick (still remembered for his Schick test, which detected immunity to diptheria) noticed that the dark-red roses his maid had placed in a vase had quickly wilted. Apparently, she then told him that this always happened to her when she was having her period, which set Schick on a path of trying to discover if there really was something powerful – or even toxic – about menstruating women.[3] Ever the scientist, Schick proceeded to carry out experiments with his maid, initially giving her and another woman, who was not menstruating, a bunch of anemones, chrysanthemums and sunflowers, and instructing them to walk around the garden holding the blooms.[4] After just a short walk, Schick observed that the maid's bunch were already beginning to wilt, spurring him on to further tests that included taking samples of his maid's armpit sweat and blood, and testing the effect of these on flowers and plants, and also on dough. His results were apparently contradictory, but nevertheless he reached a confident conclusion: *yes* – something mysterious and poisonous was definitely coming out of menstruating women's skin.

So confident was Schick, in fact, that he published his results in a Viennese medical journal, and even gave the substance a name: 'menotoxin'. Science and folklore then rather unusually found themselves in a positive feedback loop, backing each other up repeatedly and allowing the menotoxin theory to really take hold. In the early 1950s, Harvard researchers Olive and George Smith injected menstrual blood into a number of small animals, concluding that it was poisonous because it killed them.[5] (In fact, it was bacterial contamination of the blood that did so.) Menotoxin went on to be further researched and discussed in scientific journals – including the prestigious *Lancet* – all the way up to the 1970s,[6] with one study even speculating that the toxins could be having an effect not just on jam, bread and flowers, but on women themselves, and causing mood changes. The degree of confirmation bias in this story is exemplary. By all reports, every single study into menotoxin proved inconclusive, and yet there was something about the idea of periods that persuaded perfectly rational scientists to ignore the facts and reach the conclusion that most resonated with their personal hang-ups. And this deeply held sense of alarm at the thought of the polluting effects of females is by no means confined to bearded twentieth-century white men. We can find examples of 'menophobia' – an irrational fear and distrust of periods – throughout many cultures and eras in history, and reflected in our own culture to this day.

The role of all major world religions in the negative PR around periods can't be understated. With the notable exception of Sikhism, every single one of them has imposed restrictions on menstruating women, and every single one of them perceives a woman on her period to be 'ritually unclean'.[7] In Orthodox Judaism, any physical contact between a woman and her husband is prohibited during the seven days from the start of her period, a time referred to as the 'niddah', at the end of which she may become 'ritually clean' by immersion in the 'mikvah', a type of ritual bath. Christianity seems to have more hang-ups around sex than menstruation itself – but nevertheless they have the same book of Leviticus in the Old Testament, which is also found in the Jewish Torah and states that both a woman and anyone who touches her during her period are 'ritually unclean'. Some Orthodox branches of the Christian Church also bar menstruating women from sex, holy communion and touching the Bible, and in the Russian Orthodox Church, her gaze is believed to negatively affect the weather.

Islam, Hinduism and by association Buddhism also all have rules restricting women on their period. The Quran describes menstruation as an 'impurity', and Islam forbids menstruating women from touching the Quran, entering the mosque or having sex. Muslim women on their period are also exempt from daily prayers and fasting; for example, during Ramadan. Hindus are banned from entering temples during their period, and also from cooking – and touching pickles or the sacred basil plant, which some believe a woman on her period can kill simply by letting her shadow fall on it. Buddhists are fairly pragmatic on paper, seeing it as a 'natural physical excretion, nothing more, nothing less', but in practice, due to the crossover influences of Hinduism, women are often prevented from entering temples during their period, and there are some interesting beliefs, too; for example, that a menstruating woman will attract ghosts, because, as everyone knows, ghosts eat blood. In the West, some jokingly refer to women's periods as 'Shark Week' – the Buddhist ghost story seems to be the spiritual equivalent of this. Only the Sikhs – a comparatively new religion, having been established in the fifteenth century – have no restrictions around menstruation, with their founder, Guru Nanak, openly condemning the idea of seeing women as 'impure' while on their periods. This appears to be part of a wider respect for women, whom Sikhs see as equal to men. Their central scripture states: 'So why call her [women] bad?

From her, kings are born. From woman, woman is born; without woman, there would be no one at all.'[8]

Unfortunately, this kind of progressive thinking seems to be the exception, not the rule, and the idea of menstrual impurity and the need to isolate, ban and generally keep your distance from a woman on her period can be found across the globe. In many parts of the world this has real impact on the everyday lives of women and girls, with one in ten girls in Africa missing school during their periods due to both poverty and stigma, according to UNESCO.[9] And in Nepal, the ritual practice of *chhaupadi,*[10] under which periods are seen as impure, sees women and girls sent to menstrual huts, often made from mud or sticks, and windowless, where temperatures are dangerously cold in winter and swelteringly hot in summer. In spite of the Nepalese government banning the practice in 2005, it is still prevalent, and puts women at risk of death from suffocation, fire, pneumonia, snake bites and animal attacks.[11] Monica Sjöö and Barbara Mor, in their seminal 1987 book *The Great Cosmic Mother*, suggest that these practices of ostracising menstruating women were originally positive and powerful ways that women came together in female-only spaces to support each other during periods and childbirth. Sjöö and Mor see blood rituals, such as male Australian Aboriginals making cuts to their penises, as attempts by men to imitate and participate in women's blood power. Out of the same envy, patriarchal societies defined periods as 'unclean' and turned women's menstrual rites against them as a way of isolating and disempowering them. Somehow, what was once perceived as a source of power got rebranded as a source of shame – a 'curse'.

Blue Blood

The stigma of periods is deeply entrenched, manifesting both in the way they are represented in our media, and the way these representations are internalised in the psyche of every modern woman. If you are told, for example, that the best possible tampons you can buy are packaged in 'silent wrappers' that won't make any noise when you open them and alert the woman in the neighbouring toilet cubicle to the fact that you are on your period, this is a lesson in shame. Over and over again, if we look closely enough, we find periods being used to start little fires everywhere with the same messages of women's weakness and impurity.

> *'The characteristics of the powerful, whatever they may be, are thought to be better than the characteristics of the powerless – and logic has nothing to do with it. What would happen, for instance, if suddenly, magically, men could menstruate and women could not? The answer is clear – menstruation would become an enviable, boast-worthy, masculine event.'*
>
> GLORIA STEINEM, 'IF MEN COULD MENSTRUATE'[12]

Is period blood 'normal'? Pad company Bodyform decided it was, when in 2017 they became the first UK company to represent period blood not as blue, but red, with the hashtag #bloodnormal.[13] US company Kotex followed suit in 2020, with Sarah Paulsen, their creative and design director, telling the *Wall Street Journal*, 'Blood is blood . . . there is nothing to hide.'[14] The *WSJ* headline took a tongue-in-cheek approach: 'Kotex decides women's blood is red, not blue', they jibed. To repeat, this was 2020. It's funny to think how many of us sat there for decades watching the adverts show us blue liquid. How did we explain it to ourselves? We may not even have consciously considered it. But somewhere, a voice, loud or quiet, within each woman watching, must have concluded: 'They are using blue liquid because the reality is too much for people to take. The red version is a bit . . . disgusting.'

Of course, we were lucky to be seeing period adverts at all – they were banned from US television completely until 1972, and there's a taboo around not just the visuals, but the words, too, with *Friends* star Courtney Cox – then just 21 – famously being the first to say the word 'period' on a Tampax commercial in 1985,[15] and Kotex seeing a ban for their tampon ad in 2010 because it used the word 'vagina'.[16] And, along with many other realities of women's lives, such as childbirth, pubic hair, breastfeeding and body fat, period blood has been banned from Instagram, most notably in a post from Rupi Kaur in 2015, which showed her lying on a bed in her tracksuit, facing away from the camera, the slightest mark of period blood on her clothing and sheets.[17] Kaur railed against the ban, stating that it only served to prove the point she had been trying to make – that our culture will happily allow countless images on social media of women being objectified, but takes immediate offence at the sight of our menstrual blood. While pornographic images show women as the passive object, posing only to serve the male gaze, Kaur's image showed, as she put it, 'a bridge between this universe and the last' – an almost spiritual process that contains all the power of creation, which we are most often taught belongs to a male God. 'I bleed each month to help make human kind a possibility,' says Kaur. American feminist Judy Grahn isn't having the shame and stigma either – she points out that the blood of violence can be seen everywhere in our society, whereas, 'Menstrual blood is the only source of blood that is not traumatically induced. Yet . . . this is the most hidden blood, the one rarely spoken of and almost never seen except privately by women, who shut themselves in little rooms to quickly and perhaps disgustedly change their pads and tampons, wrapping the bloodied cotton so it won't be seen by others.'[18] While the blood that has become so commonplace and acceptable in our world is the blood of war, violence and death, this menstrual blood that we have been taught to feel so much shame for is, in fact, a source of power and life.

Whether you see your period as sacred or profane doesn't really change the impact that the stigma of menstruation can have on every woman's life. A 2022 survey of 1,000 women from biometrics company Forth found that only 19 per cent felt comfortable discussing period symptoms with their GP.[19] Period product company Always, alongside the charity Plan International, surveyed young people in the UK between 2015 and 2020 and found that 85 per cent of girls have tried to hide their period from those around them, while two in five reported being shamed or teased because of their period.[20] Further data from Always shows that, globally, 52 per cent of girls lose confidence at puberty and that their first period marks their lowest point in confidence during their teenage years, with 41 per cent reporting feeling ashamed and embarrassed.[21] Much of this shame and stigma finds its way into our language; just as we may find ways of avoiding naming female body parts, such as the vagina and vulva – in particular in front of children, but often in adult company and with health professionals, too – by using euphemisms such as 'tuppence', 'flower' and 'down below', so, too, with periods we seem to struggle to name them directly, speaking instead of 'getting the painters in', being 'visited by Aunt Flo', 'the time of the month' and 'the curse'. In fact, there are apparently over 5,000 euphemisms worldwide for menstruation, and while they may indeed be poetic, imaginative and even funny – 'riding the cotton pony', or, if you're French, '*Le beaujolais nouveau est arrivé*' – they are all born out of the same shame and stigma as the blue liquid and the rustle-free wrappers.[22] Even the terms we use for period products, often expressed in the signage over the relevant aisle in the supermarket – for example, 'Feminine Hygiene', or 'Sanitary Protection' – have embedded in them the idea that a period is something 'unhygienic' or 'unsanitary'. In fact, there is nothing unhygienic about period blood – it is no more germ-ridden than any of the other blood in our bodies, or for that matter a juicy rare steak. If you have a blood-borne disease, then yes, it can be transmitted via your menses, or menstrual blood, but otherwise, it's not toxic, dirty or polluting in any way.

Seeing Red

As well as being given a lifetime of gently persuasive messaging encouraging us to think of ourselves as malodorous and possibly even toxic, in particular around the time of our periods, women are also repeatedly given the falsehood that our menstrual cycles make us ever so slightly unhinged. Rarely mentioned in this discussion is the fact that, if you are on the contraceptive pill, you don't actually have a cycle at all, because you don't ovulate. So if you are on the pill and are getting mood swings, these are nothing to do with your 'cycles' – they are side effects of the contraceptive drugs you are taking.[23] For those who are not on the pill, it's true that hormonal fluctuations throughout the month can affect our moods and emotions in a variety of ways. From the higher energy many women experience around ovulation, to the tangible frustration and rage we can feel in the week before we menstruate – known as pre-menstrual syndrome (PMS), or pre-menstrual tension (PMT) – this aspect of being female can at times be weaponised against us and used to discredit us. I'm going to bet that every woman reading this has had this experience: you raise a legitimate concern about something that's bothering you – maybe at work, maybe at home – and you speak quite clearly and powerfully, and somebody makes the joke, 'Ooh, time of the month, is it?' There is a whole genre of alleged humour built around women's monthly mood swings, allowing everyone from male stand-ups to blokes in the pub a free pass to roll their eyes about women's built-in craziness in a way that wouldn't normally be considered acceptable. This can often happen at times when a woman is 'angry' or really expressing a view in an assertive 'don't-even-bother-arguing' kind of way. At the time of writing, I conducted a poll on X (formerly Twitter) asking whether women had ever experienced their feelings or opinions being discredited or undermined by suggestions that they were linked to their period.[24] Two hundred and seventy women responded: just over half of them thought that this had happened 'often', with a further 40 per cent saying it had happened 'once or twice'. Only 10 per cent said they felt this had 'never' happened to them. When I asked the follow-up question, 'If you answered yes, did you feel this was fair or justified?' just over 80 per cent responded: no.

Sometimes as women we don't challenge these situations because it can be easier to go along with the joke, and maybe, over a lifetime, we've even absorbed these negative stereotypes about 'crazy hormones' and accepted them as fact. But, while the hormonal changes of the cycle can undoubtedly affect us, there is actually no evidence that all women simply lose their grip once a month. It's true that there are diagnosable 'pre-menstrual disorders', such as pre-menstrual dysphoric disorder (PMDD – a very severe form of PMS) and pre-menstrual exacerbation (PME – where existing disorders are worsened by hormonal changes). These disorders are complex and, although hormone-related, under-researched and seem to have other contributing factors. For example, women with PMDD often have a history of significant stress exposure or trauma,[25] or sexual abuse.[26] However, the majority of women do not experience major cycle-related changes in mood, cognition or behaviour.[27] In a world in which women continue to report feeling that they have to shoulder an unfair percentage of the burden of care work and the 'mental load' (being the key person in charge of organising in the family), it's quite possible that part of the perception of PMT or PMS is women simply intermittently raising their legitimate concerns, and that hormones are just being used as yet another way to dismiss and ignore them.[28] Given that we spend around 50 per cent of our cycle either 'pre-menstrual' or 'menstruating', there's a high chance (well, one in two, actually!) that either we or others could perceive any anger or frustration we happen to express as being related to our periods, when in fact this is just a coincidence. For those women who do struggle with PMS, stress during the previous month has been found to cause it to be more severe,[29] and trauma and abuse in early life can also be a contributing factor – researchers have found that women reporting the highest levels of emotional abuse had over two and a half times the risk of PMS as those reporting no emotional abuse, and that those reporting severe childhood physical abuse were twice as likely to experience PMS as those with no history of such abuse.[30] A history of sexual abuse can also contribute to PMS, and women with this experience may also find the build-up to periods, and menstruating itself, more difficult, because of the connections between the body parts involved, the physical sensations of menstruation, and their trauma.[31] There are clearly some difficult conversations we are not having when we dismiss the emotional and psychological aspects of the cycle, and incidentally, this happens in pregnancy and birth as well, which can also be triggering events for women with a history of abuse.

Each month, between menarche and menopause, all women who are not on hormonal contraception experience a cycle, a journey through a weeks-long matriflux that reflects the wider, ever-changing matriflux of life in a female body. This makes us different from men, who don't have a monthly cycle, and don't experience other seismic physical changes during their lives such as pregnancy or menopause. It's worth remembering that, although we can see this constant shapeshifting as an inconvenience, it may only seem this way because we live in a world largely built by people who don't experience it: men. The structure of most people's work lives, for example, is built for consistency: a five-day week, week in, week out, the same – but this is not how females work: we are cyclical beings. But in a world built for the non-cyclical, periods are historically something that women have had to deny or hide in the workplace, with the underlying idea that to be successful in a man's world, we have to be like them. But this is changing, as instead of trying to make themselves fit the world, women are now beginning to shape the world to suit them, and even ask if there are aspects of the cycle that, rather than holding them back, could give them an advantage. A growing number of women's business coaches, for example, will help women in business 'harness the power of their cycle' and use tools such as charting to structure their working life around the matriflux. Dr Mindy Pelz, author of the bestselling *Fast Like a Girl*, worked with the singer LeAnn Rimes to shape not just her diet, but her entire touring schedule around her hormonal cycle. 'We need to bring the feminine back into healthcare,' Pelz told the *Feel Better, Live More* podcast.[32] 'What a lot of women are doing is just the same thing, powering through – "I'm a woman, see me roar, I can do it all month long" – and I want to point out, actually you're not designed to do it all month long.' And the spotlight is on sport, too: in 2022 Olympic medallist Dina Asher-Smith sparked conversation calling for more research into how the menstrual cycle affects women's performance in sport. 'People don't always talk about it either because you see girls that have been so consistent and there is a random dip,' she told BBC Sport. 'Behind the scenes, they have been really struggling, but outwards everybody else is saying, "What's that? That's random." I feel like if it was a men's issue, we would have a million different ways to combat things, but with women, there just needs to be more funding in that area.'[33] Later that year, over fifty female athletes joined the #SayPeriod campaign, calling for more openness in the language around menstruation in sport,[34] and Wimbledon dropped the dress code for all-white undershorts to allow female players to 'focus purely on performance'.[35] In 2024, US football star Megan Rapinoe led a new campaign, Sport Your Period,[36] to open up space for girls and women to talk about their periods and how having them affects them in sports: 'A lot of girls feel embarrassment around their period or that it's taboo. It should *not* be taboo. It's normal; it's how we all got on this earth, how we reproduce,' she said. Research into the impact of tuning in to the menstrual cycle in sports continues – one 2025 study, for example, looked at women's reaction times during their cycle, and found that, whilst some phases like ovulation had slightly improved reaction times, women bias against their own perceived ability during certain times of their cycle was not always borne out by the research results . . .[37] The conversation has well and truly opened up.[38]

Even if we are not a Grammy Award-winning singer or elite athlete, there are benefits for everyone in paying attention to their cycles. Historically, and even now, there persists the idea that the only merit in cycle charting is if we are trying to conceive, but there is much more to cycle awareness than fertility. One mindshift some women find helpful is to begin to see the menstrual cycle as part of other cycles in nature, linking it to the lunar cycle, the cycle of the seasons, the cycle of day and night, and the cycle of life itself. Through doing so we can begin to get a sense of what each 'season' is like for us, both the positives it has to offer as well as the drawbacks we have been taught to be familiar with. Cycle charting is easy and can now be done with one of a range of apps, or, if you prefer, an old-school paper and pen. All you need to do is make a note each day of where you are in your cycle and how you feel, and if you pay attention to your vaginal fluids, you may start to notice how they change when you ovulate – your fluids will usually be stretchy and slippery at this time, rather like raw egg white. Once you've worked out when you ovulate (and you may also start to notice the physical sensation of ovulation, too; a light twinge on one side), you will also have a much stronger idea of when your period will come, because the time between ovulation and your period starting is fixed – it's always between twelve and sixteen days, only deviating from this guaranteed time window in very rare cases. If you're on the pill or post-menopause, you can still chart your physical wellbeing and your feelings through each month – there is always a positive advantage in getting to know ourselves. Tuning in to our own rhythms and becoming familiar not just with our patterns, but also with our needs has a value that goes far beyond our reproductive function. At a greater level, listening to our bodies, observing their detailed activities, recording them, and talking about them openly – this is all a counter-cultural and subversive act of resistance in a world that wants us to feel shame or disgust and keep our blood hidden from view.

Red Threads

Regardless of who raised us and how we feel about them, all women have a 'red thread', or 'mother line'. This is the 'maternal' branch of our family that goes back, first to your mother, then to her mother (your grandmother), and then her mother . . . and back and back and back through time. You can think of it like Russian dolls, a long and repeating pattern of grandmothers, mothers and daughters. There is also a scientific basis to the red thread: mitochondrial DNA. This part of human DNA was the first significant part of our genome to be sequenced, and is passed directly down the maternal line of the family. Through this mother line, more is passed on than we could possibly know or imagine. If you have had any relationship at all with your birth mother, then you can already probably start to think about what she may have passed on to you. Likewise, if you have daughters of your own, you can contemplate in turn what you are passing on to them. From the trivial (facial expressions, little sayings, ways of moving, habits, likes, dislikes, recipes) to the impactful (relationship patterns, self-esteem, attitudes and prejudices, and trauma), we are all influenced by our mothers. If you have never had any contact with your genetic mother, then your red thread will be woven from both your DNA and from the influence of the woman who raised you – and the women who in turn raised them. If you were raised primarily or entirely by a male, you might like to consider whether you know anything about your mother or grandmother, or about any other significant women in your life as a child, and in what ways, if any, they may have influenced you.

It's clear that the wider culture has a lot to answer for in terms of messaging about our female bodies, but while the culture provides the scenery, it's our close family members who deliver the script. From birth onwards, most of us spend time in the presence of a woman and listen to both her direct advice and her throwaway comments about menstruation. We see the products she uses, and where she keeps them. We watch her journey through each monthly cycle. We hear how she speaks about her period, the words she uses, the tone of voice. We may hear her speak about childbirth, too, or even see her experience pregnancy and birth. And at some point, we usually have her as the key figure we turn to for information about 'the facts of life', and reassurance when we experience our own 'menarche' – or first period.

How we are taught about our first period, and how our menarche is treated by our close family, can set a blueprint that we take forward into our sex lives, our pregnancy and birth experiences, our self-confidence, and even our menopause and older years. We can hear their echoes or feel their aftershocks when we stand naked in front of the mirror, or when we are about to push our babies into the world, or when we come to teach our own children about puberty. Essentially, they can set the tone for whether we view our female body as a source of pride, something that 'works' and that we can rely on, something powerful, or instead as something weak, something that will inevitably fail us, or worse still, something disgusting and dysfunctional.

We seem to be spectacularly bad at talking to children and young people about periods. In a 2017 survey, nearly half of girls (44 per cent) said that they did not know what was happening to them when they got their first period, with a majority feeling scared and embarrassed.[39] This doesn't seem to be improving over time, either, with 76 per cent of 16- to 24-year-olds reporting that they find school lessons about puberty awkward compared to only 70 per cent of the over-fifties who took the survey. And yet, given the power that the messaging we receive about periods can wield, we should probably be placing much greater emphasis not only on ensuring that young people are informed about the practicalities of menstruation and puberty, but also on the 'origin stories' we are potentially passing on about what it means to be female. Our own origin stories came from our mothers and grandmothers, our school teachers and even the 'Tampax Lady', as she was called at my own school (we could have a whole conversation here about how and why we were entrusting menstrual education to a sales rep, but, hey, it was the Eighties!). And now it's our turn to pass on origin stories to the next generation of females. This offers both a somewhat daunting responsibility and a great opportunity – to consciously think about what we are passing on and, in doing so, try to break any negative cycles once and for all. We can do this by simply reflecting on our own experiences, and deciding what was helpful and what was unhelpful in the narrative we ourselves received. In other words, which parts of our red thread do we wish to keep in place for the next generation, and which do we feel we would like to unpick and let go of?

One simple message that it would certainly be transformative to pass on is that periods are just one small part of the menstrual cycle. Information about periods that children receive at school usually has a lot of focus on the bleed itself, why it happens and the products to use. This seems to me another way in which the male body as the 'default' is reinforced. The female body is framed as 'very much like the male apart from the disadvantage of bleeding once a month'. But to be female is very different – we have a lifetime of the matriflux, which, you could argue, requires us to be adaptable, resilient, introspective, insightful and strong. Understanding this gives us an aspirational vision of the female as she power-dances through life, cycling in connection with nature, creating, nourishing, shapeshifting and reinventing herself in response to every change and challenge.

It feels almost controversial to suggest that being female is something to celebrate. But in spite of the stigma attached to periods both historically and cross-culturally, there are, paradoxically, many examples of the rite of passage of menarche being honoured in other cultures. For example, in Japan, a daughter's first period is celebrated with a special meal of *sekihan*, made with rice and red beans. In South India, in a ceremony called *Ritu Kala Samskara*, young girls are given a party, with flower garlands, gifts and a special outfit to wear for the first time called a 'half-sari'. In some cases, it may be the case that these celebrations have their origins in a kind of 'biological essentialism' and focus on the female's capacity for reproduction as key to her worth. Nevertheless, we can take the idea of celebrating menarche forwards without having to imply that women's only value is as baby-makers. In our family, I gave my eldest daughter a little silver moon necklace that I bought for less than £10 to mark the occasion – this is also not about creating yet another commercialised event, but simply a way of reconsidering womanhood as a privilege rather than a curse.

As we reframe the female body in this way, we encourage body confidence, body literacy, self-respect. With this respect comes a deeper listening. Our bodies become something to tune in to deeply, and to take seriously. As we begin to lean in to our cycles rather than simply 'tolerate a monthly bleed', we can also begin to build a picture of what is 'normal' for us, and notice when something is not right. Periods are such an important signal of our overall health that some people call them 'the fifth vital sign' – changes in our periods or ongoing problems can be a warning sign that there is something in our body we need to address. Because period problems are extremely common, they are often accepted as normal, or something women should just put up with. However, periods should not, for example, be extremely heavy or painful, and if they are, it's important to both check in with a doctor and pay some attention to our wider health and self-care. Tiredness, stress, poor diets, under- or over-exercise and as yet undiscovered underlying health issues can all have an impact on our cycles. Women are often prescribed the pill as a first port of call if they have problem periods, which does not 'fix' anything but simply masks any issues. The pill is often prescribed for endometriosis, for example, a painful condition caused when cells similar to those in the lining of the womb grow in other places, such as the ovaries and fallopian tubes. Endometriosis is so poorly understood, in spite of affecting one in ten women globally.[40] There is currently no cure, the causes are unknown, and it takes UK women an average of eight years to get a diagnosis.[41] While the pill may alleviate symptoms in some women, it takes us no closer to understanding why this condition is happening or what can be done to prevent it. The female body is often saying, 'Something is wrong,' and being met with a shrug or, worse, being completely ignored. If we begin to listen to and respect our own bodies at a personal level, this may lead to some much-needed respect and listening at the collective level.

Blood Rites

'If you think you are emancipated, you might consider tasting your own menstrual blood – if it makes you sick, you've got a long way to go, baby.'

GERMAINE GREER, *The Female Eunuch*

Germaine Greer wrote these words in 1970 and yet they still have the power to shock. In some ways, our cultural drift in the subsequent five decades has been further and further still from the reality of our sexed bodies, as the internet has seen us rehome our consciousness in more virtual spaces, and rites of passage such as childbirth and even death have become more and more medicalised and therefore distant and intangible. If we don't want to menstruate at all, we can now take the pill permanently, according to some advice. If we do menstruate, tampon use can keep us largely at arm's length from our blood. If we've taken on board cultural and familial messages that periods are disgusting, then it may suit us to distance ourselves as much as possible from the reality of this female experience. But there is another option – to get up close and personal with period blood, and through doing so, find ways to break the intergenerational cycle of shame, and initiate healing in our own relationship to the female body.

For some women, the process of becoming better acquainted with their periods has happened almost by accident, as a side effect of their use of a new period product, the menstrual cup, which became popular in the first two decades of the twenty-first century. Motivated by the reduced cost and the environmental benefits, many women made the switch to using these silicone cups – which sit inside the vagina and catch your menses – only to discover a bonus they might not have predicted: that using the cups helps you get to know, and even start to appreciate, your period. 'I thought having to empty my cup might be the thing that put me off using them,' Abi Blake, who has been a cup fan since 2015, told me. 'But what I discovered was that my period blood was actually really interesting, maybe even beautiful?! Each day I noticed changes in colour and texture. It was actually pretty cool to be able to get up close to it and see it in a way that, although

I'd been menstruating for about twenty years at that point, I'd never really been able to. I was surprised how much I liked it.'

The artist Jenny Lewis had a similar experience. 'One day, when I had some blood on my fingers after emptying my cup, I started to wonder about why society framed up menstruation as something disgusting,' she said. In 2012, she worked with her photographer partner to create a series of images entitled 'Beauty in Blood', pictures of her own menstrual blood making shapes as it's dropped into water, which she hopes 'communicate that menstruation is nothing to be afraid of'. Lewis is one of a number of artists who explored menstrual blood in the 2010s. Liv Strömquist's 2017 series of drawings 'The Night Garden' on the subway in Stockholm caused controversy with their black-and-white sketches of women complete with leg hair and vivid red period blood.[42] Casey Jenkins caught the attention of social media in 2013 with 'Casting Off My Womb', a twenty-eight-day project in which she knitted a scarf from wool she inserted in her vagina, including during her period. Rhine Bernardino created the 'Regla Series' in 2017, a series of glass vessels filled with her menstrual blood. All of these women followed in the footstep of artists who had experimented with menstrala (menstrual art) in the 1970s, most notably Judy Chicago, who shocked the world with her 1971 image 'Red Flag' of a hand removing a bloody tampon from a vagina, and Leslie Labowitz, who was almost expelled from the Otis Art Institute in LA in 1972 for her installation 'Menstruation Wait', in which she invited onlookers to watch as she waited for her period to start. All of these artworks have the shared aim of challenging the stigma of the female body by exposing it to the light: 'The female body is leaky; it has breast milk and menstrual fluids. These are all things that are in opposition to the male body,' as Jenny Lewis puts it.[43]

Claire Baker, who has grown to love her own period so much she now works as a 'menstrual coach', told me that she has tried a variety of methods to break down her own stigmatic relationship with her blood. 'I definitely had some beliefs about my blood that it was dirty or gross or smelly or [there was] something wrong with it. So firstly I experimented with rubbing my blood on my skin – for example, in the shower. I really liked seeing it on my skin and being intimately connected with it. When I started using a cup, I liked smelling it, touching it, playing with it, making art with it. [Doing this] in a curious, playful way has helped me to realise, it doesn't smell – at all. It's really cool, the texture is interesting, it's a part of me, it's beautiful. It didn't feel weird for me at all, it felt natural to explore it.'

Other women like to put their blood to use – watered-down period blood makes great fertiliser for house plants,[44] while others use it as a monthly face mask, claiming the rich content of stem cells leaves their skin glowing.[45] There is also the option of what some call 'Blood Magic',[46] incorporating menstrual blood into ritual, either with the intention of directly healing shame around the female body,[47] or simply just to harness its power in other areas of life.[48] Claire Baker, for example, uses the contents of her cup for 'manifestation' – setting intentions alongside a ritual of pouring her period blood onto the earth. She does this as one aspect of working closely with her whole cycle, using a journal to set intentions, make plans and hopefully see them come to fruition as she journeys through each month.

You may wish to do none of these things. For some, the idea of 'period positivity' is extremely challenging; a lifetime of thinking and feeling a certain way cannot always be changed overnight. Undoubtedly, though, changing our relationships to our periods is an act of resistance. It is a refusal to accept the age-old story that our monthly blood makes us toxic, unclean, weak, insane. It's a reclaiming of the truth that periods are emblematic of women's creative power. To accept them or even love them is to accept and love the messy reality of life in the female body, and through doing so, to accept and love the messy reality of the human condition itself. The fact that so many of us hate our periods, and so many of us also hate our physical bodies, is not a coincidence.

For me, it wasn't making art or tasting my own blood, Greer style, that changed both my relationship to my menstruation and, along with it, my female body. Instead it was an experience sometimes described as 'the biggest period of your life': the post-birth bleed known as 'lochia', which lasts several weeks. There was something about the exquisite smell of my newborn, the euphoria of being free from pregnancy, the post-birth high ('I did it! I'm alive!') and the daily experience of caring for my own postnatal body as I healed that imprinted a positive memory of lochia on me. After that, each menstrual period was a sensory reminder both of those precious postnatal weeks, and of the power of being female – the gateway not just to any old new life, but to the new lives of the people I now loved the most. Those early days of postpartum are a time when many women will tell you how good it feels to 'have their body back'. Part of this is certainly the relief of literally not having a tiny human trapped in your innards any more. But it's also something greater – an almost-overnight lifting of the intense scrutiny of pregnancy, a time when your body is truly no longer your own in every possible sense.

Chapter 3

Creator Myths

'I do not wish [women] to have power over men; but over themselves.'

MARY WOLLSTONECRAFT, *A Vindication of the Rights of Woman*

Three women are sitting in a hospital waiting room; let's call them Woman One, Two and Three. Woman One is there for a meeting with healthcare professionals to discuss her plans to give birth at home. She has always wanted to be a mother, and longs for the moment when her much-loved baby will be placed in her arms. Woman Two is there for a very different reason: she has made up her mind never to have children, so she's here to consult with a doctor about the best way to ensure she absolutely never becomes pregnant under any circumstances. Woman Three, like Woman One, is also pregnant, but she feels very differently – she does not want this baby, and is here for a termination. How does the story of each woman make you feel? Do you support them all? Unequivocally? Or do you find yourself wishing to persuade one or more of them that they are making a choice that they may later regret?

In writing about childbirth, I've discovered how emotive each of these women's stories and choices can be, every one of them capable of triggering their own online debate, fuelled with anger and outrage. In each situation – birth choices, sterilisation and abortion – there will be people willing and ready to judge and even condemn women on the basis of their decisions. I've given my fictional waiting-room group the rather blank names of Woman One, Two and Three for a reason – because they are 'Everywoman'; they could be from any background or class, nationality or ethnicity. And as Everywoman, they are also interchangeable – with a different life path or set of circumstances, each of them could easily find themselves in the other's shoes. In spite of this, in the collective imagination they are often characterised as markedly different types of people, pitted against each other as if they share nothing in common and would all perhaps despise and judge each other just as they themselves are despised and judged.

Perhaps they represent something deeper, the powerful archetypes of virgin, mother and whore that embody the different dimensions of womanhood that the world finds so difficult to reconcile as parts of the same whole. First suggested by Freud, the Madonna–whore complex is based on his observations of male patients who split women into a binary of saints and sinners, unable to accept and integrate the existence of both identities within one individual. 'Where such men love they have no desire and where they desire they cannot love,' as he put it. Woman Three with her unwanted pregnancy may be our whore or fallen woman, lusty and immoral, while Woman Two may in some ways represent the Madonna or virgin, rejecting sex – or certainly its loftier purpose of procreation – completely. Woman One is the mother, an archetype traditionally associated with nurture, and also with self-sacrifice, nobly setting aside her own needs for those of the next generation. But the mother can also be an uncomfortable embodiment of the saint/sinner binary – she may be placed on a pedestal as the Madonna, but at the same time, her motherhood itself may signal her earthy powers of fertility and seduction. This unease with the mother archetype is part of the reason why we have male 'banter' or insults about how 'your mother loves it', or the stereotype of the MILF, the 'mother I'd like to f***'. It's also why we have a long history of pregnant women concealing their pregnancy under loose-fitting clothes or even avoiding being seen in public entirely, particularly during the early- and mid-twentieth century, a taboo sensationally broken by Demi Moore's naked and pregnant 1991 *Vanity Fair* cover.[1] Even the word 'pregnant' used to be avoided, with even the late Queen Elizabeth II apparently considering it to be 'vulgar', and euphemisms such as 'in the family way' used instead.[2] The mother archetype is disruptive to patriarchy because it represents the vast, multi-dimensional reality of the female: we are strong, soft, capable, vulnerable, fertile, creative, sexual, sensual, maternal and powerful. We are the matrix – a word that today means the origin point and epicentre of development or creation, but which, as we know, has its roots in the Middle English word for womb.

Patriarchy attempts to tame and control this disruptive, multi-dimensional matrix in a variety of ways. Rather than being irreconcilable archetypes, in reality Woman One, Two and Three are united by the same challenge: the desire for their own reproductive autonomy, and the realisation that they are almost certainly going to have to fight for it. Woman One, pregnant and wishing for a home birth, will have her choices scrutinised by everyone from the person next to her in the supermarket queue to her healthcare professionals. She will be given mixed messages, on the one hand told she is free to choose where and how she has her baby, on the other hand finding that her freedom of choice is narrowed by everything from the availability of midwives to her personal health and risk factors. Women who choose home birth recount a long list of spurious reasons they are given to discourage them, from their BMI, to the 'mess', to the fact that they rent rather than own their home.[3] I can remember, when I planned a home birth with my own first child in 2008, being told by midwives that the stairs in my house could cause a problem, because they were 'too narrow for a stretcher'. The terrifying image of me being so incapacitated by childbirth that I had to be stretchered out of my house lodged in my brain and kept me awake at night, while in reality the chances of such an outcome were undoubtedly miniscule. Nearly twenty years later, news coverage about home birth is often littered with references to 'risk' and 'danger', in spite of UK NICE guidelines supporting it as a safe choice for low-risk women.[4]

But please don't think this is simply about home birth. Women's birth choices face scrutiny no matter what they want, whether that's elective caesarean, epidural right from the start, zero pain relief or freebirth with dolphins. There is something about true freedom of choice in childbirth that makes even those who claim to support it nervous and confused, in particular the freedom to make what others perceive to be 'bad' or 'wrong' choices: a 2013 study published in the journal *BMC Pregnancy and Childbirth* perfectly encapsulates this conflict, with the professionals surveyed agreeing that on the one hand, 'women were the ultimate decision makers', but on the other hand stating that 'the needs of the woman may be overridden for the safety of the fetus'. The Atwood quote always springs to mind: 'A rat in a maze is free to go anywhere, as long as it stays inside the maze.'[5] Birth freedom is an illusion and only applies to those women who make choices that meet the approval of her current culture and period in history.

If Woman One pushes buttons because of her 'selfish' wish to prioritise her own birth experience over perceived risks to her baby, Woman Two, clear about her lack of desire to ever be a mother, is arguably even more likely to induce outrage and moral panic. Women asking for sterilisation surgery, known as tubal ligation, or 'having your tubes tied' – in particular, younger women who have no wish to have any children at all – are likely to be met with a flat no by their doctors. Olivia Downs, from Massachusetts, sparked debate in 2022 with a TikTok that has since had over half a million views, telling the story of a visit to her gynaecologist at the age of 22, asking to be sterilised.[6] 'No, it's permanent,' she was apparently told. 'And you might meet Mr Right and change your mind.' In response to Downs, women from around the world shared their own similar stories, and their sense of frustration that they were living in a country that had just rolled back its abortion rights with the overturn of *Roe v. Wade*, and yet didn't seem to want women to be sterilised either. 'It's like they don't understand a kid is kinda permanent also,' as one commenter on Downs' video put it. Since abortion rights were rolled back in America, tubal ligation rates in women aged 19 to 26 have increased by 70 per cent,[7] with one woman sharing her procedure on a viral TikTok with the comment, 'Getting sterilized because y'all couldn't act right in the voting booth'.[8]

Even women who have already had multiple children may be discouraged from the procedure. Charlotte Baker from Somerset had had three children by the age of 28 and met with resistance when she asked to be sterilised: 'I was adamant I didn't want any more, but they weren't happy about it. They kept saying, "But what if you meet someone else and want to have kids with them?"' she told me. 'I was made to see three different doctors, and was told the last one would "talk me out of it". She didn't, she agreed. I'm 37 now and it's still the best decision I've made.' Some women, such as Pia Ryan from London, were never able to find an amenable doctor. When she asked to be sterilised at 31, she had already had children but was met with a flat no. 'I'm a woman who knows how to make decisions with conviction,' she told me. 'I pursued my request to the level of senior consultants and was repeatedly told that I was too young and may want more children in the future, so ever since then I've had to take the pill instead. I feel the medical profession is woefully sexist. I did not change my mind and I am now 49. I knew what I wanted.'

Not all women who decide never to have children ask to be sterilised – but they usually still face a backlash. Globally, birth rates are falling, in many higher income countries well below the rate of 2.1 babies per woman needed to keep a population stable.[9] The reasons for this include better education and access to contraception, but another leading factor is choice: women are collectively deciding against marriage, monogomy and children. When influencer and model Ellie Gonsalves shared 117 reasons for not wanting to have children in 2023, these included everything from world overpopulation to losing her figure.[10] She was praised by some for her honesty, but she also received 'hundreds of DMs telling me how much of a horrible and broken person I am'.[11] The flip side of increasing numbers of women deciding to be 'child-free' are the 'pronatalists' – championed by Elon Musk and supported by Trump and JD Vance – a movement claiming concern for the future of humanity but heavily tinged with right wing conservative values alongside fears of the immigration that may be needed from lower income countries if populations dwindle.

And Woman Three? Well, the global fight for women's right to free, safe and legal abortion worldwide is well documented. Abortion laws vary from country to country, but figures from 2021 show twenty-one countries, including Malta and Andorra in Europe, Iran, Egypt, Laos and Madagascar, where abortion is illegal in any and all circumstances. More than fifty other countries have tight restrictions on when abortion is permitted, relating to the physical and sometimes mental health of the mother being at risk, while others permit it only in the case of rape, incest or foetal abnormality. There is no country in the world where abortion can be accessed with no restrictions whatsoever – even the most moderate have regulations around gestational time limits, most commonly set at twelve weeks.

And, of course, in June 2022, the Supreme Court in the US overturned the landmark ruling of *Roe v. Wade*, removing the constitutional right to termination, leaving the rights of women across large swathes of America damaged and uncertain. Just as the female body itself is seen as untrustworthy, so, it seems, are women's autonomous choices.

In countries where abortion is restricted, women are impacted in a number of ways, some more starkly visible than others. In Poland in January 2021, a near-total ban on abortion was introduced, and in September of the same year,[12] and January of the following, two different women died of sepsis, both as a result of a doctor's hesitancy to intervene and terminate pregnancies that were not viable.[13] Since the overturn of Roe v Wade in the USA in 2022, several women have died due to lack of access to abortion, including Amber Thurman in Georgia and Josseli Barnica in Texas, who both died of sepsis after their access to healthcare was restricted and denied.[14] Their stories echo that of Savita Halappanavar, whose death in Ireland in 2012, also due to sepsis from pregnancy complications, sparked international protests and a march of around 12,000 people in Dublin demanding the repeal of the Eighth Amendment, a piece of Irish law that gives the mother and foetus equal rights to life. The repeal they fought for was granted in 2018, although the legacy of the interweaving of Church and State in Ireland pervades. The impact of any culture that sees the rights of the unborn as equal to the rights of the woman who carries it will not just be felt by people seeking a termination. Its effect seeps into all areas of women's bodily autonomy: the disregard for their body boundaries sees them treated simply as a means to an end – for example, by forcing them to give birth by caesarean if they are thought to be making unsafe choices, as happened with Adelir Carmen Lemos de Góes in Brazil in 2014.[15] Even in the throes of labour itself, they are told that others need to make decisions for them or that they are not the 'expert' on their own bodies: one woman who gave birth in Ireland in 2015 told me she was informed, 'You will give birth when, how and where we decide.' When she questioned their decisions they said, 'Clearly someone has to be the voice for your baby since you are not being very rational.'

Whether the baby is wanted or unwanted, if the accepted belief enshrined in law is that the foetus is of equal value with the living, breathing mother, then it inevitably follows that women will be expected to sacrifice their own bodies, needs or even their lives for an entity that depends upon them for its very oxygen. Women become, as two different US senators termed them in debates about abortion in 2017 and 2019, 'host bodies', and the foetus, with its equal rights, is thought to have 'personhood'. Prior to the fall of *Roe v. Wade*, laws that gave personhood before the line of 'viability' – the time in gestation around twenty-four weeks when the baby foetus can survive outside the womb – were banned. This didn't stop at least thirty-eight states having foetal homicide laws, which categorise the foetus as a potential crime victim, leading to several hundred women in the US being prosecuted and even jailed for pregnancy outcomes such as miscarriage or stillbirth. And now, post *Roe*, anti-abortion activists are calling for laws that give the legal protection of 'personhood' to the foetus before viability, or even to embryos. This could mean child endangerment laws being applied to the foetus, with a wide and devastating impact on everything from what a woman eats or drinks in her pregnancy, to whether she is legally compelled to delay life-saving treatments such as chemotherapy. IVF treatment and the freezing of embryos could also be affected, as could access to contraception such as the IUD (coil) and the morning-after pill, both of which could prevent the implantation of a fertilised egg and therefore violate personhood.[16] Women and their bodies, it seems, must be controlled even at a cellular level.

The cellular is the personal is the political is the cosmic. A person fighting against the rights of Woman One, Two or Three to birth at home or be sterilised or have their pregnancy terminated, or even for the right to life of a newly fertilised egg, may feel they are embroiled in a discussion about one individual's choice, but in fact, they are caught up in what I sometimes think of as 'star wars' – not the movie, but nevertheless an intergalactic struggle of cosmic proportions, in which never-ending different groups of teeny-tiny and only mildly effective spaceships try in vain to shoot down the vast and limitless energy of . . . what shall we call her? Mother Earth? Grandmother Spider? Gaia? Sheela na Gig? The Great Cosmic Egg? The Matrix? However we name it or envisage it, this huge and powerful creative energy appears again and again in stories and myths from every culture, in particular the ones that try to explain how the world first began – and if you ever give birth, you may feel it pulsing and vibrating through your own body, just for a time. It's so massive and so powerful, and while sometimes the instinct is to admire or worship it, more often our patriarchal world seeks to covet it, take credit for it, control it, impersonate it or even destroy it. An individual woman having her bodily autonomy denied will be deeply affected, but in the grand scheme of things, it's just the millennia-old *pew-pew-pew* of the little spaceships, firing off their bullets, which mostly bounce off the infinitely powerful Feminine.

Origin Stories

> *'She shall be called Woman,*
> *because she was taken out of Man.'*
>
> GENESIS 2: 23

One way of sending out little *pew-pew-pews* is by simply writing a narrative in which the most powerful type of person is male and then making sure that narrative is spread far and wide. There's a meme that does the rounds on social media of a woman holding a placard at a feminist protest that reads: 'I didn't come from your rib, you came from my vagina.' It's funny because it's a reversal of the biggest lie ever told: the two largest world religions, Christianity and Islam, both teach that Eve was made by a male God out of Adam's rib. The idea that the first woman was born from a man's body is obviously the complete opposite of what we all know to be reality, but it's certainly an effective way of setting out the stall of patriarchy and positioning men as the ones with the most important power of all – the power to create. Even when Eve does give birth to her first child later in the book of Genesis, the Bible tells us she says, 'With the help of the Lord I have brought forth a man.' This Eve – to blame for temptation, sin and the Fall from paradise, and condemned to be 'ruled over' by her husband and experience painful childbirth – has definitely got things off to a terrible start for the Sisterhood. And her story, still told to little boys and girls around the world today, reinforces the idea of 'Woman' as weak, secondary, powerless and culpable. How many little girls who hear it must feel that, given the choice, they would rather be Adam?

The idea that the power of creation belongs to men is by no means confined to religion. Another story you may well have learned in school is that of the heroic sperm's epic journey or 'race' to fertilise the egg. In fact, if you go on to Google right now and do an image search for 'cartoon sperm and egg', you will find illustrations of this, perhaps reminiscent of your teenage biology lessons: the egg is depicted wearing lipstick, perhaps with a flower in her hair, batting long eyelashes and gazing coyly at the sperm, who is shown flexing his biceps, wearing cowboy hats or superhero capes, and looking cool in sunglasses. The sperm is 'active' – he will get the prize of the egg if he is the strongest and fittest and wins the race, while the egg is passive, and simply waits for her hero to arrive. Just like Eve, the egg is a character that 'things happen to'; she is a supporting actor in the story. Creation is not her business.

This story – of action-hero sperm and passive egg – illustrates brilliantly how the patriarchal desire to claim the territory of creation is written into our understanding of our very biology. In fact, anthropologist Emily Martin was the first to recognise how, linguistically at least, our conception story betrays our social assumptions about gender roles, in her 1991 essay *The Egg and the Sperm: How Science Has Constructed a Romance Based on Stereotypical Male-Female Roles*.[17] Now, thanks to recent advances in understanding, science has caught up with Martin's critique: the egg is not passive at all. She has her own journey – and if we want to create a narrative of winners and losers (which, arguably, is also quite patriarchal), then she is also a winner. The female ovaries contain little sacs, called follicles, where there are always eggs in different stages of development. Each month, around ten of these follicles start to get bigger and stronger, and if you wanted to frame the story this way, you could think of this as a competition – which follicle will become dominant and release the winning egg?[18] Imagine them all, wearing sunglasses and vest tops and pumping barbells in their little training follicles, and then, suddenly, one of them triumphs, and with one last flex of her biceps, pops out of her follicle and is taken up by the fallopian tube. The fallopian tube, by the way, is another part of female reproductive anatomy that 'does stuff' – rather than just being a highway from the ovary to the uterus, the fallopian tube has 'fimbriae', finger-like projections that catch the egg as it is released.[19] How do they do this? They are lined with hair-like structures called cilia and, at ovulation, they move in closer to the ovary and beat the cilia in rapid motion, sweeping up the egg into your fallopian tubes. Which, as you might recall, are named after a man – sixteenth-century Italian anatomist Gabriele Falloppio.

The egg could be thought of, then, a bit like the sperm, as active and strong, as a winner. OK, OK, I hear you say, but once she's in the fallopian tube, she waits for her hero, right? Not so. Without the egg, the sperm would, quite literally, be lost – because it's progesterone, released by ovarian cells, that stimulates the sperm and attracts them towards the egg. This chemical signal from the egg causes sperm to be 'hypermotile' – stronger and wrigglier and, basically, better swimmers.[20] Without this, sperm would lack the strength to reach and fertilise the egg. And there's more: scientists are now beginning to understand that the egg may actually play an active role in choosing which sperm to attract.[21] In a process known as 'cryptic female choice', the egg's follicular fluid gives off chemical signals that can influence which sperm are selected and therefore able to reach them. In a study on mice, it was shown that the eggs showed a preference for sperm from less-related males. In humans, studies have shown that different eggs will have different preferences, with some eggs being better at attracting sperm from one male, while a different egg from a different female was better at attracting sperm from a different male. All of these relatively recent discoveries about the role of the egg have surprised scientists. Professor Daniel Bryson, the senior author of the 2020 study that showed this microscopic selection process, said, 'The idea that eggs are choosing sperm is really novel in human fertility.'[22] This novelty may at least in part be down to the male-centred narrative that humans have for so long superimposed: even at a cellular level, we have assumed the male is more active, dynamic and powerful.

And it's not just the egg that plays a part in conception – the female body works in a variety of ways to ensure that only one sperm cell with intact DNA makes it to the egg.[23] The vaginal fluids, which if you're female you may have observed are more slippery and stretchy around ovulation time, become thinner, less acidic, and also greatly increase in volume – you'll produce around ten times as much fluid on fertile days as on other days of your cycle – all allowing sperm to move better and live longer in the vagina. But your vaginal fluid can be hostile to sperm, too – in a similar way to the egg's follicular fluid, it will also filter out sperm that have a closer genetic profile to your own.[24] Your cervix may then play a role in selecting the fittest sperm: it contains tiny grooves which the sperm swim up, and those with abnormal shapes don't travel through the grooves as easily, getting flushed back out by the vaginal fluid. And, if and when a sperm does make it past the mighty egg's rigorous selection process, then she has a few finishing tricks – including initiating a reaction in the head of the sperm to allow it to fuse with her outer matrix,[25] known as the 'zona pellucida', which it does by gently 'spooning' with her, according to developmental biologist Scott Gilbert – a process of 'melting together', rather than the violent penetration that is often described.[26] Once this has happened, the egg then quickly pulls up the drawbridge, so to speak, by changing the structure of the zona pellucida so that no further sperm can gain access.[27]

Every story you are told about the female body, even if it's presented as 'science', bears further scrutiny. Even as I've researched the last few paragraphs, I've had to search extensively to discover more about the female role in conception, with so many articles and pieces of research written with the sperm always playing the protagonist and the egg barely getting any of the lines.[28] It's reminiscent of the many film's that fail cinema's Bechdel Test, which states that there must be at least two female characters and that they must talk to each other about something other than a man. And then there are the possible 'myths', one of which I heard being propagated on BBC Radio 4's *Woman's Hour* in 2023 – that the female orgasm plays a role in conception, too, with the waves of physical contractions causing a kind of 'upsuck' that draws semen deeper into the female body. At first glance, this might seem like a feminist piece of info: 'Stop Press: The Female Orgasm Is Important!' But, of course, the 'upsuck' effect only makes it important if you position conception, rather than women's pleasure, as the main purpose of sex, which, when you think about it, is a pretty retro idea, with strong links to religious ideals. In fact, from Hippocrates all the way to the eighteenth century, the belief that female orgasm was essential for procreation allowed religion to approve of and even encourage female pleasure. But once it started to become clear that artificially inseminated animals – and women – could get pregnant with zero pleasure at all, there began a growing unease around the mysterious female orgasm, and the emphasis shifted to its use as a cure for 'hysteria', fuelling a highly lucrative industry for doctors and early vibrator manufacturers. And there is an unpleasant flipside to the idea of the orgasm causing a beneficial 'upsuck': at my Catholic school in the early Nineties, I remember being told by an anti-abortion group who came in to give a talk that 'you can't get pregnant if you are raped, because the body tenses up'. This was echoed as recently as 2012, when Todd Akin, a member of the US

House of Representatives, sparked outrage during a discussion about abortion by saying that 'from what I understand from doctors, pregnancy after rape was rare [because] the female body has ways to try and shut that whole thing down'.[29] This is, of course, nonsense, and damaging nonsense at that, with the female body being given a role in defending itself against violation and therefore some of the burden of responsibility if this mechanism, as Akin put it, 'didn't work'. In this event, he said, the rapist should be punished, but not the foetus. This is not a new idea: in medieval times and antiquity, and even as recently as the early nineteenth century, a pregnancy could potentially result in a rapist's acquittal, because, 'without an excitation of lust, or the enjoyment of pleasure in the venereal act, no conception can probably take place'.[30] The stories we tell about the female body often seem to say more about us, our perspective on women, and in particular our desire to claim authority over them, than they do about actual biology.

The Hostile Uterus

Throughout the eighteenth century and for much of the nineteenth, the thoughts and imagination of the pregnant woman were thought critical to how her child would eventually look. In order for the child to resemble the father, the mother would have to think the 'right' thoughts. A child who did not resemble the father, or a sick or disabled child, was invariably the fault of the mother's immoral mind.[31] We may not have understood very much about pregnancy and conception, but nevertheless, we perceived the female body as potentially hostile. If you're reading this and you've been pregnant in the twenty-first century, this eighteenth-century idea that a mother's body, rather than being a place of nurture, could instead cause damage, might resonate with you. When I was pregnant for the first time in 2007, I had a few cravings, not for lumps of coal or banana on my pizza, but for everything on the extensive 'banned list' – I wanted what I was 'not allowed': a rare steak topped with a runny egg, followed by a plate of blue cheese, all washed down with a large glass of red. But, without much explanation as to 'why', I was told I must avoid these things, and this seemed to be congruous with the much wider messaging I was picking up that my body was no longer fully my own, and that I could not therefore be trusted to make the correct decisions about it. As someone who, up until that point, had casually assumed that the work of feminism was largely done, it came as a bit of a shock. People touching or commenting on my 'bump', sometimes even strangers, seemed to encapsulate this same energy, which was presumably why I – and I know I'm not alone here – found it infuriating. The explanation was always, 'Oh, they are just being friendly, they are so excited and happy for you!' etc., but their actions seemed metaphorical for society's sudden sense of ownership over my body – something I had always believed belonged to me alone.

The advice can differ greatly from country to country – if you're in England, you'll be advised to avoid the sauna,[32] but in Finland you will be positively encouraged to enjoy its health benefits, for example.[33] Generally speaking, recommendations don't seem to be built on very robust evidence, due in part to the fact that randomised controlled trials with pregnant women would not be considered ethical. Advice over the years has changed – that runny egg I craved in 2007 is now back on the UK menu, as long as it's produced under a scheme like 'British Lion', which apparently makes it less likely to contain salmonella. How much the risk is therefore lowered, and what the actual risk is to your baby if you *do* get salmonella or any other form of food poisoning during pregnancy, is not usually part of the information given to women and can be difficult to establish. The economist Emily Oster, pregnant herself and movitated by her own love of coffee, decided to investigate food advice for her 2013 book, *Expecting Better*, discovering, to nobody's great surprise, that many of the restrictions are based on absolute worst-case scenarios, the majority of which are incredibly unlikely. For example, the chances of getting listeria from an unpasteurised blue cheese, according to Oster, are something like 1 in 8,000, and even if you are unlucky enough to get it (and you can also get it from foods that are not on the banned list), the chances that serious harm will therefore come to your baby are even smaller.

'Worry is the work of pregnancy.'
PAM ENGLAND, *Birthing from Within*

Oster has come under fire, though, in particular for her advice on alcohol in pregnancy. Although she is clear that very heavy drinking in pregnancy is bad for your baby, when she researched *Expecting Better* she could find no evidence from the data that low levels of alcohol consumption were a problem. In 2016, the UK Department of Health updated their guidelines, stating that no level of alcohol was safe in pregnancy, having previously suggested that women could have one or two units, once or twice a week.[34] But this update was not based on any new evidence, but rather a concern by doctors that, even though one or two small drinks were unlikely to be harmful, pregnant women might underestimate the amount of alcohol they were consuming, and that it was therefore safer to take a black-and-white approach.[35] In other words, women couldn't be trusted and, rather like children, needed a clear and firm parenting style that their developing brains could fully understand. This attitude isn't only applied to alcohol – current UK guidelines also suggest that you limit herbal tea to four cups a day. There doesn't seem to be any evidence for this, nor any stories of ill effects, unless you are talking about a specific tea, and even then you might as well be saying 'limit salad intake' because there are such a variety of herbal teas and each one would require its own study. Nevertheless, they confidently picked a number of acceptable cups and stuck it in the guidelines anyway.

Whatever you decide to do in pregnancy, your choices may well be scrutinised and judged in a way that you are not used to, but which will absolutely follow you into motherhood. Pregnant women have reported being refused service in the local coffee bar,[36] and humiliated when asking for a glass of wine in the pub.[37] If you think the barista or the barman was right to do this, how would you feel about a mother being prosecuted if she did cause harm to her foetus by her pregnancy choices? This question has been tested in law: in 2014, a case was brought to the English Court of Appeal in an attempt to prove that the mother of a baby born with foetal alcohol syndrome committed a crime under the Offences Against the Person Act 1861, and that the child was therefore deserving of criminal injuries compensation.[38] The case was significant, with over eighty more children with possible claims for compensation apparently waiting on the outcome. The court ruled that no such offence had taken place, but essentially, what the court was debating was whether or not the foetus could be considered, in the eyes of the law, a 'person'. Intervening in the case were both pro-choice organisation the British Pregnancy Advisory Service (BPAS), and anti-abortion lobbying group the Pro-Life Research Unit, and both knew what was at stake here. In the US, anti-abortion groups have used similar cases to erode women's autonomy, because if you can get a ruling that suggests the foetus is a 'person', you can begin to police pregnant women's choices and behaviours. The female body becomes dehumanised; an area to monitor and mistrust, a potential crime scene or even a murder weapon.

Such attitudes, whether enshrined in law or not, can become a destructive part of a pregnant woman's psyche. The idea that the female body can be a harmful place for a baby to develop is most powerful to those women who suffer miscarriage or stillbirth, or whose babies experience health problems. Were they somehow to blame? Women will often forensically examine their behaviour in the wake of such events – were they wrong to keep up their fitness class? Should they have had such intense sex? Did they get too hot? Too cold? Was it something they ate? Even if they have been following all the guidelines, they will still work hard to find a way to find themselves guilty, in situations where, most often, the usually bossy voice of 'science' suddenly goes quiet, leaving a void for them to fill by offering no explanation for their loss or their child's difficulties. During the coronavirus pandemic, uptake of the Covid vaccine was slow and hesitant, and again, women were blamed – why would they not just take the doctor's advice? But as Clare Murphy, then CEO of BPAS, pointed out, we were expecting women to take something unknown into their body, having repeatedly reinforced the idea that everything from herbal teas to salami was potentially unsafe without much clear research to back up the diktats. 'We have created a climate where women are expected to avoid any possible risk to their pregnancy even in the absence of any good evidence of harm,' she said in 2021. 'The challenges we are seeing with the Covid-19 vaccine uptake are an inevitable consequence of this.'[39]

The Tree of Life

The organ that works the hardest to protect the foetus from harm – the placenta – is, in our Western culture, most often treated as clinical waste. After my first birth, nobody asked me if I wanted it, and it was whisked away and presumably incinerated. In other parts of the world, this organ, sometimes referred to as the 'tree of life', because of the trunk and branch-like pattern that its system of veins creates, is treated with more reverence and respect. In New Zealand, the Māori call the placenta *whenua*, meaning 'land', and it is buried, along with the umbilical cord, in a significant place.[40] This is considered important to reinforce the relationship between the newborn child and the land of their birth. Some see the placenta as having human attributes, most often those of a sibling or twin, while others feel it to be significant in other ways.[41] In Ancient Egypt it was thought of as the child's secret helper, while in Cambodia, it is believed to be the origin of a person's soul and is buried surrounded by spiky plants to keep away intruders. Many believe the handling of it directly affects how the child will grow up – in Indonesia, for example, it is often placed in a pot with symbolic items such as a pencil and paper to encourage intelligence, a mirror for a bright and clear personality, a razor blade for clear speech, money for prosperity and a thread for long life. This pot is then often thrown into the sea if the child is a boy, to encourage travel and adventure, or buried by the house if the child is a girl, to encourage her to stay at home and raise a family. Inspired by some of these stories from other cultures, I kept the placenta of both my second and third children and buried them under a tree we had planted when my first child was born. The first time we did it, my partner heroically dug the hole, and we both felt a bit silly in some ways, while in others it felt good to create a ceremony of sorts, in a world where we are increasingly less likely to mark significant rites of passage. I'm not married, and my children aren't christened, but I did stand in a cold and muddy field and read 'Now That I Am Forever with Child' by Audre Lorde, my 2-year-old skipping around, tying ribbons to the trees, my newborn cradled in my arms.

I bore you one morning
just before spring
My head rang like a fiery piston
My legs were towers between which
A new world was passing.

Instead of seeing the placenta as a waste product, or even something disgusting or 'hazardous', there was something intuitively right about treating it as something special, and as a part of the amazing process of pregnancy that had brought me the children I now loved. The biology of the placenta is a wonder in itself: it begins to form around a week after the fertilised egg – known at this point as the blastocyst – implants into the uterus.[42] Some cells from the blastocyst break away and burrow deep into the uterine wall, and it is these that will become the placenta, developing with the baby to eventually be quite large – around 10 inches long and an inch or so thick by the time of the birth, and weighing up to a pound. The mother's blood passes through the placenta and provides the baby with oxygen, nutrients and antibodies, at the same time acting as a filter, keeping out waste and toxins. Essentially, it acts as the lungs, liver and kidneys of the foetus, allowing a transfer to happen from mother to baby's blood, without their blood ever mixing. As well as this, it is an endocrine organ, producing hormones essential for the pregnancy to continue. Whether you appreciate the placenta at a spiritual level or not, it can't be denied that something extraordinary takes place within the female body – it is the only time a whole new and incredibly complex and multi-functional organ will grow within an adult's body, and then be expelled once its purpose is fulfilled. And yet it is also mistrusted, causing arguments throughout the ages as to how it should best be removed after the birth (clue: in most cases, it's best left to its own devices), and even today being another part connected to the female body that is spoken of in less than positive tones: 'insufficient', 'dysfunctional' or just plain 'old'. If birth is simply a mechanical process with the woman as a machine of production, then it makes sense to simply see the placenta as a 'waste product'. Rather than being celebrated, the placenta is most often mistrusted and then incinerated – symbolic of our disrespect for women, the mother, the Earth and the tree of life itself.

Forever with Child

When Audre Lorde wrote in 1968 that she was 'forever with child', she presumably meant in the sense of the permanent and unbreakable emotional connection that all parents understand; as another writer, Elizabeth Stone, expressed it, 'To have a child is . . . to decide forever to have your heart go walking around outside your body,' or as John F. Kennedy apparently more bleakly said, 'To have a child is to give fate a hostage.' In fact, those of us who have been pregnant are 'forever with child' in a way that Lorde could not perhaps have imagined: in a process known as foetomaternal microchimerism.[43] Since the 1990s, studies have begun to show that, during pregnancy, cells from the foetus pass through the placenta into the mother, potentially remaining in her body for decades. A 2012 study found male cells, containing the Y chromosome, in both the blood and the brains of women who, years before, had been pregnant with boys.[44] It is thought that microchimerism may also occur during breastfeeding,[45] and that the transfer is two-way, meaning that, as I sit here typing, my body may contain cells not just from my three children, but also from my own mother. Microchimerism happens in those pregnancies that, for whatever reason, don't make it, too. It's thought that cells can cross the placenta as early as seven weeks, a comforting thought for those who have experienced loss.[46] What function these foetal cells may have is yet to be properly understood,[47] but they have been observed to migrate to places of injury in the mother's body,[48] stimulating the healing process, and have even been found in caesarean scars. And, perhaps most astonishingly, foetal cells have been found to migrate to the mother's heart, potentially helping her to survive a heart attack.[49] However, in a way that seems more than a little metaphorical for motherhood itself, foetal cells may bring healing one day and trouble the next, potentially contributing to issues like auto-immune disorders or Alzheimer's. The science is still emerging and there is much yet to discover. For now, the idea of a little part of our children staying with us forever and even repairing our broken hearts will have to be enough.

It's not just our hearts that are affected by motherhood, but our brains, too, in ways that are only just beginning to be understood. Most of us are familiar with the concept of 'mummy brain' or 'baby brain', and may even perhaps have had it used against us at some point, as happened to me once, in the midst of an intensely serious meeting with colleagues when I was working for the NHS as a therapist during my first pregnancy. While speaking, I struggled for a moment to bring some facts to mind (perhaps I hadn't had enough coffee), and a colleague began to laugh and said, 'Ah! Baby brain!' They were a nice person, and I'm pretty sure they were just being light-hearted and certainly didn't expect me to be writing about it in a book fifteen years later. But something about it felt seismic. 'Just a joke' – but the implication that even though I was only a few months pregnant, this new-found state was already having a noticeably detrimental impact on a part of myself I probably valued above all else – my thinking power – was terrifying. It tapped into a deep-seated fear that motherhood was going to undo me; that simply by becoming pregnant, I had set myself on a path that would, in all manner of ways, make me a lesser, downgraded version of myself. As it turns out, the opposite is true, neurologically speaking at least. This is yet another body myth, yet another negative story about being female, which, once the layers are removed, reveals something positively beautiful. As Dr Sarah McKay, neuroscientist and author of *Baby Brain: The Surprising Neuroscience of How Pregnancy and Motherhood Sculpt our Brains and Change Our Minds (For the Better)*, put it to me, 'The hormones of pregnancy sculpt our brains and change our minds in preparation for motherhood. Mother Nature did not intend for pregnancy to make us stupid.' Researchers now speculate that being repeatedly told that motherhood will have a detrimental effect on our cognitive abilities is in fact planting seeds of doubt in the minds of women and making them wrongly attribute any normal memory lapse to their maternal state.[50] In addition, this negative reinforcement may actually be distracting us from the interesting truth that having a baby could actually change our brains in positive ways. Studies have found, for example, that women's brains reorganise their connections during pregnancy, essentially becoming more efficient, not just in their ability to be attuned and attached to their infants,[51] but also in their spatial associative memory – essentially that ability to remember where we put things and find our way around (all the mums reading will nod knowingly at this).[52] Interestingly, the brains of first-time mothers have been compared to those of adolescent girls, and been found to undergo similar changes – the matriflux is a neurological experience, too, it seems.[53]

Motherhood does change us. The idea that these changes will be largely negative is an easy sell when we are already fearful – of the changes in our bodies or of getting 'baby brain', perhaps, but, at a deeper level, fearful of becoming mothers in a world that does not value the mother. We carry all of these fears with us through pregnancy and then into the labour room itself, where they meet and mingle with both the individual fears of our care providers and their collective and institutionalised mistrust in the female body. Here we encounter one of the biggest body myths of all: that in spite of the fact that the majority of women can conceive and grow a baby with no external help whatsoever, the same will not be the case when they come to give birth. The raw, wild power of this experience will be tamed, measured and managed, until it is brought firmly and decisively under control.

Chapter 4

Power Myths

'In any society, the way a woman gives birth and the kind of care given to her and the baby points as sharply as an arrowhead to the key values of the culture.'

SHEILA KITZINGER,[1] WOMEN AS MOTHERS

Women may spend a lifetime feeling that their body is poorly built and somewhat unreliable, but never does this come more powerfully to the surface than in the experience of childbirth. Doubt was my first emotion when I realised I was pregnant for the first time, age 32, swiftly followed by a fear that was so dominating it followed me around for the whole nine months, stalking my days, making me tearful at random, and lurking in my 3 a.m. imaginings. I can still remember looking at my reflection in the bathroom mirror after that positive pregnancy test and staring at my body in terror. Instead of thinking, *Wow, you are going to be a mother!* my mind instead went immediately to the fact that whatever was in there was going to get bigger each and every day and then bust out of my teeny-tiny vagina.

Like many women of my generation, I had never been told anything positive about childbirth. I had watched the educational school video, which in my case was an Eighties woman with a perm, big glasses and a Laura Ashley frock lying on a bed looking like Something Very Bad was happening that she hadn't 100 per cent agreed to. I'd seen births on soap operas and TV dramas and 'The One Where Rachel Has a Baby' on *Friends*. I'd been told that when you give birth you have to let go of all your usual boundaries around who looks at or touches the most intimate parts of your body in a process so integral to the experience that it even has an official name: 'leaving your dignity at the door'. I'd been assured that when it came down to the wire I wouldn't care about the dignity thing because I'd be 'so out of it' and, anyway, 'all that matters is a healthy baby'. I would nod at this but secretly wonder why, in this experience that was supposed to be so special, I wouldn't matter, too.

Only one person during my entire first pregnancy said anything positive to me about the birth itself, and this was a mother of a friend of my partner; I didn't know her particularly well but she was one of those women who had an air of strength and capability about her. We were in an Indian restaurant in a large group, noisy and celebratory; I was probably the only sober person. She leaned in to me and said, 'Are you scared?' and pointed to my bump. 'Um, yes,' I said, expecting the rest of the conversation to be about my forthcoming dignity bypass. Instead, she just looked me in the eye and said, '*It's not that bad*.' This was new information. 'Really?' I said, incredulous. 'Yes, really,' she said, firm and convincing. 'Everyone says it's awful, but it's really not that bad at all. It's a bit like a really bad period, maybe a bit worse than that, but really, *not. that. bad*. You'll be fine.'

I clung to her words like Leonardo to Kate's raft at the end of *Titanic*. In the ice-cold sea of negativity I then found another warm current: browsing in a bookshop I happened on a copy of the brilliant *Birth: A History* by Tina Cassidy, which immediately helped me to see modern birth practices in the context of other women, in other cultures and times. Cassidy highlights the progress brought by modern medicine alongside the mistakes: '. . . medical help has often meant isolating babies in nurseries, receiving an unnecessary episiotomy, having a breast dipped in iodine before every feeding – whatever the latest trend. If only we'd known how skeptical we should have been. And still should be.' I began to question whether some of the elements of childbirth I was most afraid of – the loss of control, the instruments, the undignified rummagings in my vagina, the unbearable pain – could potentially be bypassed completely if I, Milli Hill, just 'did well' at this challenge. How had I done well in the past? By studying hard, of course! I bought more books.

Immersed in my 'Being Top of the Class at Birth' project, I discovered the work of pioneers like Ina May Gaskin and Sheila Kitzinger, and devoured them. Here was a counter-cultural narrative, suggesting that birth was something powerful and celebratory; as Kitzinger puts it, it's 'not something we suffer, but something we actively do and exalt in'. Gaskin had attended hundreds of births in her Tennessee commune, the Farm, and she seemed convinced that the female body was fit for purpose: 'Your body is not a lemon,' she writes. 'Human female bodies have the same potential to give birth as well as aardvarks, lions, rhinoceri, elephants, moose, and water buffalo. Even if it has not been your habit throughout your life so far, I recommend that you learn to think positively about your body.' This was the feminism I had been searching for, all tucked away in the pregnancy section of the bookshop and told with the same capable humour as my friend's mum in the curry house. 'There is no other organ quite like the uterus,' Ina writes in her *Guide to Childbirth*. 'If men had such an organ they would brag about it. So should we.' The message from Gaskin, Kitzinger and other pioneers like Janet Balaskas, who created the idea of 'Active Birth', seemed to be that rather than being weak and passive, women really could 'do' this thing themselves, and that it might even be positive, or empowering. This wasn't dissimilar to the messages women of my generation had been given about other areas of our lives – we didn't need a man to help us, supervise us or control us; we could lead, we could be successful, we could 'have it all'. In the birth room, too, the idea appealed that, rather than being helpless and in need of rescue, we could actively birth our baby, and even catch them with our own hands. Sisters were doing it for themselves: our bodies, as well as our careers and relationships, were areas where power could be reclaimed.

Like many women both before me and after me, I marched confidently into my meetings with midwives and consultants with a sense of my rights, only to find that the 'system' hadn't really got the memo. They didn't seem to have read Cassidy, or Kitzinger, or Gaskin, or Balaskas, but were instead firmly entrenched in the idea that women's bodies in childbirth were deeply unreliable, and that there was nothing they were doing to make this situation worse – quite the opposite! They were rescuing women on a daily basis from the fate that would surely befall them if their female bodies were left to their own devices. Walking into your obstetrician's office in 2007 and asking if you could discuss alternatives to hospital birth or induction or indeed anything slightly different to the standard offering was a bit like walking into your boss's office in 1967 and asking if there might be opportunities on the management team. It was met with incredulity at best; at worst, with scathing judgement of the sheer audacity of having such wild ideas above your station. However, in the obstetrician's case, the systemic paternalism was considered, and still is considered, entirely justified because the belief is so embedded that the female body in childbirth is something unreliable or even dangerous, far too hot for women to handle.

When someone is afraid they are much easier to control. As the reality of these power dynamics began to dawn on me, my first pregnancy became a quest that went beyond the personal. Were they right? Was there something about the female body that meant we could not be relied on to give birth? Were all these interventions – the monitoring, the inductions, the episiotomies, the forceps, the caesareans – necessary? Should women accept them with gratitude, lie back and think of England, and let their dignity be lost amid the panic and chaos of this extremely risky event? Were the likes of Gaskin and Kitzinger feminist gurus? Or potentially deadly mavericks, encouraging women towards 'natural' experiences that put them in unnecessary danger? I pursued these questions almost forensically over the following years, through my first birth, which ended with some of my biggest fears being realised (induction, episiotomy, forceps), and my second, where I faced those same fears all over again, sitting in a pool of water at home and crying with panic until suddenly, there she was, and I had done it. And then my third, during which I convinced myself that the second one was a fluke; again, I sat in a pool of water at home overbrimming with doubt, until suddenly, there he was, and again, I had done it. These three births punctuate a decade during which I started a global movement to try to use the burgeoning tool of social media to improve childbirth for all women, no matter what kind of birth they wanted or ended up with, and wrote a bestselling birth book with the same aims. At the same time, in my own world of sleepless nights, nappies, Mumsnet and toddler groups, I met woman after woman who had been damaged by her birth experience, sometimes physically, but most often emotionally and psychologically. They were sad, hurt, disappointed. They had felt scared, abandoned, belittled, unheard, unsafe. They had hoped for a positive or empowering experience, but instead it had been traumatic. Some of them could not face a second baby. Many of them blamed themselves, feeling they should not have got their hopes up. These personal experiences reflect what has been described as an 'international public health problem', with as many as 45 per cent of women experiencing a traumatic birth globally.[2] As I made playdough or soothed a crying baby at my breast in the small hours, I wondered, was this part of our lot as women? Or could it be different?

For some women, it *was* different. Like the women I had read about in Gaskin's *Guide to Childbirth*, I came across women in my own life who spoke of birth as a rite of passage, a transformative moment in which they were more connected to their power than ever before or since. Such women describe feeling like a goddess, roaring like a lioness, exploding in constellations of fireworks and comets, encountering ancestors, and connecting to some kind of universal super-grid as they travel to the stars and bring back their baby. For them, birth is a kind of epic, massive experience, during which they are forever changed. These women are extremely rare, but I became one of them, with my second and third home water births. Nobody touched me during those births. Not once, except perhaps my partner to hold my hand or my little 2-year-old who came to kiss me and bring me a bunch of hedgerow flowers as I floated in my watery nest. Cow parsley, buttercups, red campions – when I sit in my chair in old age I will remember that bunch of flowers as one of the most exquisite moments of my life. Why do I get to have that memory, though, while other women have to endure horrifying flashbacks of experiences they wish they could erase forever? Why did my female body manage to give birth in that way, but theirs did not? Are we different?

The short answer is no. The long answer is, it's complicated. We do benefit from modern medicine in the birth room, there's absolutely no doubt about that. Even under the care of Ina May Gaskin herself, there are some women who will need interventions: of the nearly 3,000 women who gave birth at her birth centre, the Farm, between 1970 and 2010, fifty of them needed caesareans, and 148 needed to transfer to the hospital.[3] But that's a caesarean rate of under 2 per cent, when in the US this has risen from 5.5 per cent in 1970 to at least 30 per cent or higher today,[4] and in England in 2024–5, 45 per cent of births were via caesarean, meaning it overtook the numbers of women having a spontaneous vaginal birth for the first time in history.[5] Much lower caesarean rates can be found not just at Gaskin's commune, but from other similar models of care; for example, the renowned Albany Midwives who ran from 1997 to 2009 in Southeast London, serving an 'all risk' caseload in an area of ethnic diversity and social deprivation (all factors thought to lead to higher rates of intervention), had a caesarean rate of 16 per cent; or the Lismore Birth House in New South Wales, Australia, which also served 'all risk' women in the mid-2010s and had a caesarean rate of 6 per cent.[6] In spite of these outcomes, such models of care often come up against significant pushback from those who deem them unsafe: at the Albany, for example, midwives were accused of dangerous practices and it was eventually shut down.[7] In all of these models of care, two key things happen which distinguish them from the mainstream: the woman and her midwives have time and space to build up a relationship, and huge attention is paid to female physiology and the needs of a labouring woman. In other words, birth outcomes have very little to do with the woman herself, and an awful lot to do with how she is cared for and treated.

Birth in Captivity

In the early 2010s, I wrote a weekly column for *Best* magazine about all things birth. My pieces were most often hooked onto celebrity stories, and in the summer of 2013 my editor, the fabulous Abigail Blackburn, asked me to write about a celebrity with a difference: Tian Tian, the giant panda. Abigail had noticed that in all the news reports about preparation for the panda's possible birth in Edinburgh Zoo, great care was being given to making sure the panda was as undisturbed as possible.[8] Visitors were redirected away from Tian Tian's enclosure, she was monitored only by CCTV, a special 'cubbing box' had been built and extra insulation added to her enclosure to keep out noise. When it came to pregnant pandas, as I wrote in my column, we understood clearly just how much their environment could affect them – so why did we not afford the same consideration to labouring women? And could it be that if we did, we would find that fewer interventions were needed?

In the modern birth room, we place women in busy, high-tech environments, often brightly lit and unfamiliar. We build the birth space around the needs of the care provider – beds so they can easily examine the woman, bright lights so they can easily see, doors that swing open so they can come and go, tools and technology in view so that they are easily to hand. But none of these things would wash with Tian Tian. As a mammal, she needs to feel quiet and safe in order for her birth to proceed as it should. If we did not give her this safe, undisturbed environment, and she then had complications in her birth, we would quite rightly blame ourselves. Somehow, though, we seem to feel that human beings are able to override this mammalian nature, perhaps for the simple reason that we like to think of ourselves as superior to pandas. And when we don't give women what they need in labour, and their births are complicated, we very quickly blame, not the system, but the woman. Her female body is somehow not able to give birth without assistance.

All mammals in labour have similar hormonal processes and similar needs. Cat, dog, chimp or panda; most will seek out an undisturbed location in which to give birth, knowing that the process of labour makes them and any resultant tiny offspring particularly vulnerable. In early labour, stress or fear can trigger the release of catecholamines – the hormones such as adrenaline that are responsible for our 'fight or flight' response – causing labour to stall or shut down completely. Many women notice this effect when they make the journey from home to hospital, only to find that the disruption of a car journey or the bright lights of the busy corridors seem to have had an impact on the strength and frequency of their contractions. Whether we regard the car trip or the labour ward as 'safe' at an intellectual level, our mammalian hormones may decide otherwise. The production of adrenaline or beta-endorphins in response to stress may inhibit the production of the key hormone of labour, oxytocin – and the modern response to this is often to give the woman a synthetic version of this hormone via a drip. This will be described and written in the medical notes as 'failure to progress', often understandably perceived by women to be a judgement that their faulty bodies let them down, when in fact a labour that slows or stops in response to the woman's environment, waiting until she has found the optimal conditions for her birth, could instead be held up as an example of the female body working exactly as it should to keep both mother and baby safe.

'Failure to progress', commonly cited as the leading reason

for unplanned caesarean sections in many countries, including the US, Australia, and the UK, is also often measured against a graph, sometimes known as 'Friedman's Curve'. Developed in the 1950s by Dr Emanuel Friedman of Columbia University, the concept behind this graph or 'partogram' – that the cervix will dilate neatly at a machine-like rate, most often 1 cm per hour – is still widely used today as a yardstick of the expected progress (or lack of it) of the female body in labour. More recent studies, such as an important one by Jun Zhang in 2010, have challenged some of Friedman's findings, but not his underpinning ideology that there is an ideal template for the progress of labour, which can and should be charted on a graph.[9] Added to this, like much of modern childbirth research, the women being measured are all giving birth 'in captivity' – or, if you wish to put it more gently, in unnatural situations that would definitely not be considered optimal for Tian Tian the panda. In Zhang's study, for example, all of the births were in US hospitals, half of the women were given oxytocin to speed up their labours and 80 per cent had epidurals.

The Body Versus the Clock

For a childbirth culture based around the speed of cervical dilation, you need two things: a clock, and regular vaginal exams. The former features so heavily in most modern labours that some US hospitals have large digital clocks on the wall. Cynthia Overgard, hypnobirthing expert and host of the *Down to Birth* podcast, told me how her nearby hospital in

Connecticut even 'pushes a button' on the clock when the woman is admitted, and that they are told by the doctor, 'I'm going to need to see you dilate at a centimetre an hour, so you have to have the baby within ten hours,' regardless of how long they have been in labour before attending the hospital. 'I've also heard that when women reach ten centimetres in that hospital, they reset the timer, and women are told, "Two hours till C-section."' To monitor this 'progress', regular vaginal exams – when a doctor or midwife inserts fingers into the vagina to measure how dilated the cervix is – are essential. These exams, which in most Western countries are performed routinely every two to four hours, are often experienced as invasive and undignified, and although they are completely optional, it is not unusual to find women who have no idea that they can decline, or who realise they can but nevertheless lack the confidence in their own bodies to do so.

This creates what academic midwife and author Rachel Reed calls a 'cervical-centric birth culture', in which 'the body is conceptualised as a machine with distinct parts that can be broken and understood separately . . . The woman has disappeared,' and is replaced instead by a diagram and measurements.[10] This dehumanisation and reduction of women to a single body part is epitomised by some of the language around birth stories; for example, 'I was only two centimetres,' or 'Room Five is fully dilated.' The cervix is also pictured in the minds of both care provider and birthing woman as a sort of mechanised circular opening, dilating like the doorway of a cuckoo clock, while all around it remains unchanged, whereas in fact the physiology of labour is complex and it is the contractions, fired by the hormone oxytocin, that pull the uterus upwards and cause the cervix to stretch slowly open around the baby's head. The woman's entire physicality, hormonal systems and consciousness move together through labour in an intricate dance. She is more than just a container that opens, or fails to open.

As well as being invasive, even potentially introducing infection or accidentally breaking a woman's waters, vaginal exams don't have a great evidence base and are only as scientific as a pair of fingers feeling inside the depths of a woman's vagina can be.[11] Nevertheless, this inexact method is relied upon to such an extent that, in some cases, care providers will check the cervix one final time before granting the woman 'permission' to begin pushing. In other words, the woman's instinct and the feedback she is getting from her own body is felt to be even less reliable than the birth attendant's measurements. Added to this, even if the measurements are accurate, the cervix can be unpredictable, dilating at speed or very slowly, or a mix of both, or, in some cases, becoming less dilated if the woman is disturbed or anxious. Some midwives feel there are other, better ways to keep an eye on labour progress – first and foremost to rely on the woman and her own instincts, and secondly to tune in to her movements, her behaviour, her facial expressions, her sounds and even (some say) the smell of the labour room, as an indication of the imminence of the birth. Many women (76 per cent in one study[12]) will also have a purple line on their skin that extends from the edge of their anus upwards on their lower back, becoming longer as they get closer to birth. This line, which can also be blue, red, whitish or pink, and less visible in women with a darker skin tone, is not very well researched or understood, but is thought to be caused by pressure on the blood vessels in the area increasing as the baby's head descends. Another sign can be observed in the 'rhombus of Michaelis', a kite-shaped raised area on the lower back caused by a section of bone moving backwards and increasing the diameter of the pelvis. According to midwife Jean Sutton, the appearance of the rhombus also coincides with another sign – the woman's hands 'reaching upwards . . . to find something to hold onto as her pelvis is going to become destabilised'.[13] Sutton adds that the rhombus is what birth expert Sheila Kitzinger 'was talking about when she recorded Jamaican midwives saying the baby will not be born "till the woman opens her back"'. However, this specific widening of the pelvis will not happen to women who are lying on their backs, in spite of this being the most common choice of birth position for the majority of Western women.

During labour, instead of being on her back (which can narrow the pelvic opening by up to 30 per cent), a woman moving freely will make instinctive choices as she spirals deeper into the place some call 'Labour Land'. Flooded with endorphins and oxytocin, her 'thinking brain' – the neocortex – will quieten, and she will drop down into her older 'feeling brain' or limbic system. Midwife Rachel Reed has observed that women in this trance-like state will even choose positions instinctively according to the position of their baby. 'Sometimes from the outside the movements will make no sense but you have to trust they are what the mother and baby need. Only after the birth do you sometimes discover the baby was in a tricky position, which at some level, the woman seemed to know and be working with,' she told me. The majority of women, though, will not labour in this way, and will instead find that they are assumed to have so little expertise that they are kept supine and told exactly when and how to push, and in some cases, subsequently informed that their pushing time is up and that they will now have a caesarean. For women who have had an epidural, the guidance of external observers is vital, because they will not be able to feel their own contractions. But for those women who can feel them, 'coached pushing' – which has become so synonymous with births on TV that you will rarely see one without a small team of people yelling, 'PUSH! Now pant! Now PUSH!' – is often not only unnecessary, but yet another example of the erroneous messaging women receive that their bodies and instincts are unreliable.

The Valsalva manoeuvre, named after a seventeenth-century Italian physician who developed it as a method of clearing pressure in the ears, is an approach to the pushing phase in which the woman will be instructed to take a deep breath, hold it for ten seconds, and then push as hard as they can. Also known as 'purple pushing', because the resultant pressure will often cause her face to become very red or 'purple' – and, in some cases, blood vessels in her eyes to burst – it is often accompanied by phrases such as 'push into your bottom', or even (and I heard this one myself once on a fly-on-the-wall childbirth documentary) 'get angry with your baby'. There's no evidence that purple pushing has any positive effects for women, other than helping them to give birth more quickly and therefore beat the oft-imposed two-hour time limit for the second stage of labour, but there is evidence that it can be detrimental to postnatal urinary continence, and, of course, disempowering or even humiliating for the woman to experience.[14] Far worse than Valsalva, though, is another 'manoeuvre', this time named after Polish-born gynaecologist Samuel Kristeller.[15] Banned in the UK but still used in several European countries,[16] the Kristeller manoeuvre involves huge pressure being applied to the top of the 'bump' during the pushing stage. Again, this serves to both manage and control labour and hasten delivery, but in the process it can cause severe complications or even death to mother or child.[17] And if you can possibly bear to hear one more example of unnecessary damage done to women in the name of childbirth speed and safety, the episiotomy, in which the vaginal opening is made larger by a cut to the perineum, is performed as standard in many births globally, with stats varying: up to 40 per cent in some US hospitals in 2020[18]; 100 per cent in Taiwan in 2002[19]; 45 per cent in China in 2021[20]; 15 per cent in the UK and France; 72.9 per cent in Portugal in 2010.[21] Post-episiotomy healing can be complex, with the leading UK review of the evidence concluding that its routine use cannot be justified.[22]

Narrow Pelvises, Fat Vaginas

On her back as others shout at her urgently, a woman in the final throes of labour may feel completely deskilled and overwhelmed, and perhaps, as I did when I first got the blue line in the pregnancy test, that the task she faces is physically impossible. Told throughout life that giving birth is like 'shitting a bowling ball', most women will be surprised and relieved to learn that this analogy doesn't stand up to much scrutiny. For starters, a baby's head is not massive and rock hard, like a bowling ball – at 27 inches, a bowling ball is around double the circumference of a baby's head, which measures around 13.5 inches at its widest point. (To help you visualise, that's about the circumference of a standard unused loo roll). Added to this, the baby's head is probably more like that squishy toilet roll than the watermelons and pineapples pregnant women hear so much about – it's relatively malleable, with two soft spots called fontanelles where the bones of the skull are not yet fused, allowing 'foetal head moulding' to take place, with different parts of the skull overlapping in order for the baby to be born.[23] Even better, the vagina is extremely strong and, filled with little folds called rugae, is designed to stretch as big as is needed to accommodate the baby's transit. Like the allegedly 'pea-sized' clitoris, the vagina is chronically underestimated. As Ina May Gaskin puts it, 'Men take it for granted that their sexual organs can greatly increase in size and then become small again without being ruined. If obstetricians and women could understand that women's genitals have similar abilities, episiotomy and laceration rates might go down overnight.' In spite of the vagina's power, the idea that it is not up to the job of childbirth persists, with one doctor who spoke alongside me on a BBC radio discussion even claiming – with zero evidence to support him – that rising caesarean rates were due to women's vaginas getting 'fatter'.[24]

While you may not have heard the unlikely tale of the fat vagina, another, much older body myth is so readily accepted that you will probably have had it presented to you as fact at some point, and it's this: human birth is difficult because we have evolved to walk upright. Known as the 'obstetric dilemma', and first put forward in 1960 by the American anthropologist Sherwood Washburn, the theory (and it is only a theory) is that because we used to be apes but have now evolved to walk upright and have intelligent babies with big heads, we have had to reach a kind of evolutionary compromise in order to give birth. This 'compromise' basically means that female humans have had to develop the widest possible pelvises we can sustain, while remaining able to walk on two legs, and that our babies need to be born as early as possible, rendering them dependent on us for longer than primates. Not only is this the reason why human birth is so difficult and literally a great big problem to be solved, but the compromise goes beyond childbirth and suggests that, in every area, the female pelvis makes us less physically able than men. You could go so far as to say that the obstetric dilemma positions femaleness as a kind of disability.

Striding confidently forward to stamp all over this theory with her highly functional legs is Holly Dunsworth, professor of anthropology at the University of Rhode Island.[25] 'The assumption built into this is that women are already worse bipeds than men, and evolution can't allow them to get any worse,' she tells me via Zoom. 'Instead of a multitasking view that women are good bipeds *and* good birthers, instead the theory frames it that they are bad at bipedalism, and bipedalism is keeping them from being good at giving birth, too.' Dunsworth explains that it's the fact that men were controlling the narrative that tells us not just how these ideas began, but also how they have taken such hold, woven into the fabric of how people think about the story of evolution and treated as fact even by those who had never heard of the term 'obstetric dilemma'. 'The people who came up with it were men who were intensively studying the fossil record and obsessed with bones,' she says. 'In skeletons the difference in the pelvis captured their imagination. The human skeleton that develops as male was viewed as the ideal human form, and the female as like a deviant or compromise from it. The way they saw it, the men were doing these wonderful strong, swift, elegant things with their bodies and the women could just manage childbirth, but barely!'

Dunsworth looked to the work of another researcher, Anna Warrener, who had already tested the hypothesis that women's wider hips made them worse at walking and running, and found it to be, as you would probably expect, incorrect. OK, so we can walk and run, but what about childbirth? It *is* true that we're rubbish at this, right? Dunsworth is sceptical. 'The solution that must exist in order for us to "solve the dilemma" is that we give birth to our babies early, but there is no evidence for this,' she explains. Birth is a 'tight fit' in terms of size of baby and pelvis, this much is true, but our gestation is not particularly shorter than other primates, some of whom also have a tight fit at birth and all of whom also grow their brains to full size in childhood rather than in utero. Some also have highly dependent newborns. In spite of this, some researchers have even put forward the idea that human babies are under-developed at birth, extra needy and more like those of 'altricial mammals', such as rats and kangaroos, which are born in an immature state, than of other primates. I'd not heard this idea before, but as a mum of three, I'd definitely been given the impression that there was something especially annoying about human babies that made them particularly hard work. This, too, says Dunsworth, needs scrutiny. 'Who was telling these stories from the beginning? Who had the voice? It was mostly men. And their narrative of human babies – as useless, as parasites, as extra-uterine foetuses – is not a very nice one.' Human babies may be unusual and deserving of scientific investigation, but simply explaining all this in a way that denigrates not just women's bodies, but babies and the act of motherhood itself, speaks volumes about the misogyny that underpins not just scientific theory, but the mistaken distrust in the reliability of women's bodies that lingers in every labour ward. As Dunsworth so brilliantly summarises: 'Women are not "compromised" and our bodies do not pose dilemmas to be solved. We are just as adapted as men, and all the proof you need is that we birthed all of them.'

Lie Back and Think of England

Much of modern antenatal preparation, which is also often itself distrusted and considered unreliable, is focused – rather like this book – on an 'unlearning' of the negativity that many women have unconsciously absorbed about their body and its abilities. For example, women who may have only ever pictured birth on a bed on their back with coached pushing may be taught instead about the foetus ejection reflex (FER), a phenomenon that some women describe rather graphically as feeling like 'reverse vomiting', in which the body completely takes over and, without any conscious effort from the woman, pushes out the baby rapidly in just a few contractions. According to French obstetrician Michel Odent, FER will only happen if the woman is attended by a midwife who stays calmly in the background, allowing the woman to lose control of her 'thinking brain' or neocortex, and enter what Odent calls a 'quasi-ecstatic state'.[26] If, on the other hand, the birth attendants attempt to coach or 'support' the woman, FER will be unlikely, as he explains in his 2015 book *Do We Need Midwives?* 'The foetus ejection reflex can also be inhibited by eye-to-eye contact or the imposition of a change of environment, as would happen, in our modern world, when a woman is transferred to a delivery room. It is inhibited when the intellect of the labouring woman is stimulated by any rational language, for example if the birth attendant says: "Now you are at complete dilation. It's time to push."'[27]

Instead, once fully dilated and at the phase known as 'transition', the woman will experience a natural surge of adrenaline, which makes her suddenly alert and often fearful. (Often at this point a woman will say, 'I cannot do this', 'I need an epidural', or even 'I want to die' – this is adrenaline speaking.) The same 'fight or flight' hormones that in early labour can cause the process to slow, now work instead to speed it up and trigger a fast birth. If you imagine again our mammal in the wild, if her labour is just getting going but something causes her to feel unsafe, her hormones will tell her body, 'Not here, not now,' but if her birth is imminent, and she has reached a point of no return, she is extremely vulnerable and it is probably safer for her to have her baby as quickly as possible: FER is the logical solution. The accompanying surge of adrenaline also gives the mother energy both to meet and bond with her baby, and to protect it if necessary – it seems everything, left to its own devices, works just as it should. Odent believes the whole process of childbirth is hampered by our human attempts to help it: 'One cannot actively help a woman give birth. The goal is to avoid disturbing her unnecessarily,' he wrote in *Birth Reborn* in 1984.

Forty years later, and although many women, whether they realise it or not, are still being taught something of Odent's vision for birth, it slips further and further from reality. In some ways it's almost pointless for a twenty-first-century woman to learn about natural or undisturbed birth unless this comes in tandem with a full set of instructions on how to stand up to her doctors, know her rights in childbirth or make a birth plan – and then she will be mocked for these attempts to wrestle back the control and the positive birth experience that she knows is possible and rightfully hers. There are many examples of women being the butt of jokes for their attempts to have a voice in the birth room, from doctors laughing at them on X about how the length of their birth plan will correspond to the length of their caesarean scar, to a leading obstetrician poking fun at Meghan Markle at an international conference: 'A doula and a willow tree, let's see how that goes!' he jibed to much laughter from a global audience of doctors.[28] Bestselling book *This Is Going to Hurt* by Adam Kay describes a woman with a 'nine-page birth plan, in full colour and laminated', who has abandoned it and is headed for surgery. This, he says, does not surprise him: 'Two centuries of obstetricians have found no way of predicting the course of a labour, but a certain denomination of floaty-dressed mother seems to think she can manage it easily.' In 2018, Dublin-based obstetrician Aoife Mullally described women who make birth plans as 'over privileged, over-anxious middle-class "birthzillas"', who 'think they are the only woman who's ever given birth',[29] and in 2023, a US-based doctor retweeted a woman's birth plan with the caption 'This baby may not make it out of the hospital'.[30] Point out these misogynies and you place yourself in the firing line: after a decade of speaking to women about their experience of childbirth, and creating two books, three babies and an international birth organisation, I have been treated as an opinionated upstart by some: one told me a water-birth film I shared was 'propaganda',[31] another accused me of 'psychological abuse' for talking about birth as a positive experience, and on BBC Radio 2, Dr Sarah Jarvis pulled rank when I raised the issue of women feeling coerced into induction by stating, 'I've been a GP for thirty years and my experience is, the vast majority of women don't have this sort of experience.'[32] Later in the same programme, she told the story of two stillbirths she had witnessed over her long career, to support her argument that women should not object to induction – exactly the kind of coercion I had been trying to draw attention to.[33]

All of this sniggering and fearmongering works in tandem to maintain the narrative in which a woman who does try to take control of her birth in some way, but who doesn't have the experience she hoped for, ends up feeling that she is to blame, keeping hold of all the feelings of trauma and guilt herself when in fact they belong to the system that casually stacked the odds against her from the start. The idea that women would be more satisfied if they did not have such unrealistic expectations has a much wider resonance than the experience of childbirth: you will find a raft of articles, for example, if you google 'women's unrealistic dating expectations', but interestingly, nowhere near as much seems to have been written about how men should lower theirs. Essentially, the articles claim that women's higher standards – which they presumably have been enabled to have in the past few decades because they have finally been able to access education and economic independence – are 'ruining dating'. This sounds an awful lot like the 'feminism has ruined marriage' argument, or, as the Christian broadcaster and presidential hopeful Pat Robertson put it in 1992, 'Feminism encourages women to leave their husbands, kill their children, practise witchcraft, destroy capitalism and become lesbians.'[34] Lesbianism was the closest poor Mr Robertson got to mentioning sex, but it might not be too unfair to imagine that he believes women should keep their expectations low in that department, too. 'Lie back and think of England' is apparently what late-nineteenth- and early-twentieth-century women would do, having been married for economic reasons to men they did not love and who were perhaps unattractive, unwashed and unskilled in female pleasure, but it is not a great leap to see parallels between these archaic attitudes to sex and modern attitudes to childbirth. Just as sex was once considered, for women at least, to be something unpleasant or even traumatic that simply must be endured for the benefit of reproduction, now childbirth gets the same treatment: hop up on the bed, lie back and wait for it to be over. The goal in both is the 'healthy baby': the process is not something we participate in, but something that is done to us, and that we must simply endure 'for England' (or, indeed, whichever country we are contributing a new human to). In both, we are taught body myths that hold us back from our power; in both, we are taught to prioritise someone other than ourselves; in both, we are encouraged to keep our expectations low lest we be disappointed.

At some level, it is perhaps even considered crude, selfish or 'unladylike' to have a thirst for pleasurable physical experiences, in the birth room or the bedroom. Even now, in 2025, some women still find it difficult to speak about their own sexual pleasure, to ask for what they want in bed or to initiate sex – so deeply have we internalised the 'good girl' attitude that prizes restraint and compliance over lustily letting go. Interestingly, the phrase 'good girl' is used frequently in the labour ward, so much so that it was written about in the *British Medical Journal* in 2018 as an example of language that disrespects pregnant and labouring women as autonomous adults.[35] The sounds and energy of natural labour are raw and sexual; anecdotally, I have heard of midwives who prefer the quieter labour room that ensues if a woman chooses an epidural, with one memorably describing a woman labouring freely as 'unseemly'. In 1982, led by Janet Balaskas, over 6,000 people marched at a rally in London at the Birthrights rally, in protest at the lead obstetrician at the Royal Free Hospital's claims that giving birth upright or on all fours was 'animalistic behaviour'.[36] There is something about labouring women that, for some, is too wild, too visceral, too sexual, and needs to be brought back under control.

And yet, as some (most notably Sheila Kitzinger) have observed, birth *is* sexual. For a few – more than one in twenty, according to a 2016 survey – it is even orgasmic, which at first may seem a ridiculous concept, akin to 'joyful dentistry' or 'ecstatic chiropody'.[37] However, as all women know, mindset plays a huge role in sexual pleasure, and mindset can be dramatically affected by environment. You're unlikely to have great sex if you've already decided beforehand that it's going to be lacklustre, or if you don't feel like it's your place to say what you want and need. You're even less likely to do so if you're trying to get it on in a room full of strangers with the telly on and the lights up bright, or if you feel like you're only allowed to stay in the missionary position, or if someone suddenly switches on the orgasm countdown clock on the wall. The anatomy of the clitoris also gives us more information about why birth is orgasmic for some women, with the baby exerting pressure on the internal parts of the clitoris as they descend. Some women will spontaneously reach down and touch their external clitoris in labour, while others will deliberately try masturbation or some 'alone time' with their partner, because clitoral stimulation and orgasm will help stimulate the hormone oxytocin, helpful if labour slows down or stalls. One writer, Margaret Jowitt, author of *Dynamic Positions in Birth*, has even raised the question of whether the clitoris, rather than being solely for women's pleasure, actually plays a role in labour, possibly by triggering the Ferguson reflex (not to be confused with the foetus ejection reflex, this reflex, named after Canadian doctor James Ferguson, occurs when pressure from the baby's head on the cervix causes a surge in oxytocin and intensifies contractions to push the baby out).[38] Jowitt also speculates that the engorged crura and bulbs of the internal clitoris may cushion the baby's head, that it may be part of the stimulation of oxytocin needed for bonding, and that it could be the 'seriously large nerve plexus' that Jean Sutton suggests triggers the movement of the rhombus of Michaelis, widening the pelvic opening.[39] Jowitt appears to be the only person who has even raised these questions, which, like so much about the female body, remain unanswered. Instead, birth is seen through the lens of male sexuality – the whole of labour merely a build-up of pressure, to be got through as quickly as possible before the 'main event' when the baby is 'ejaculated'. But even if not literally orgasmic, the whole of labour, as well as the moment of birth itself, can be a deeply sensual physical experience, not separate from female sexuality, but part of its power. 'The same energy that gets the baby in, gets the baby out,' as some say, or as Kitzinger puts it more beautifully:

> *Her face lights up as she realizes that this is her baby being born, a living being from her body, and she can see its head and reach down and feel it as it slides into life. Suddenly she is full, stretched to her utmost, as if she is a seed pod bursting. There is a moment of waiting, of awe, of the kind of tension which occurs just before orgasm, and then suddenly the baby passes through, the whole body slips out in a rush of warm flesh, a fountain*

> *of water, a peak of overwhelming surprise and the little body is against her skin, kicking against her thighs or swimming up over her belly. She reaches out to hold her baby, firm, solid, with bright, bright eyes. A peak sexual experience, the birth passion, becomes the welcoming of a new person into life.*[40]

Pain and Power

The elephant in the room in any discussion about positive, or even orgasmic, birth, is pain. During pregnancy, it can seem the go-to topic of conversation of literally everyone from the bloke in the pub to every midwife and doctor a woman encounters: 'What are you going to do about pain relief?' If I had a pound for every time someone had said to me, 'You wouldn't have a tooth out without drugs, would you?' I'd be richer than a dentist. The short answer to this, which I have trotted out on many an occasion, is that having a tooth out (or any other kind of surgery) tends to happen when something is going wrong with the body, when there is a problem that needs to be fixed, whereas giving birth is the body at the absolute peak of its abilities and power, a healthy body in its prime, working exactly as it should. One of the problems, though, with twenty-first-century birth, is that we are often setting women up to fail, and adding in the notion of birth 'without pain relief' just compounds this. 'Are you going to give birth without pain relief? Wow! That's brave!' The reality is that no woman can give birth without any pain relief. She may decide not to have gas and air, or an epidural, but she will have to find something to replace these; for example, a birth pool, or support from a midwife she knows and trusts, or access to the resources she needs to give birth at home, or mindset work such as hypnobirthing, yoga or meditation, or the confidence that comes from knowing your options, or the ability to move freely, or a doula or other solid birth support. Just rocking up at the hospital having decided to 'go with the flow' and 'maybe not have any pain relief' might work, but on the other hand, she may find she cannot cope. Again, she will blame herself for this, thinking that perhaps other women who do manage without pain relief are made of sterner stuff. The system that fails to understand or support female physiology will again be off the hook.

Perception of pain is complex, but the basic summary is this: if you are told something is going to really hurt, it probably will. Research also shows that anxiety and fear raises our perception of childbirth pain,[41] whereas feeling that the pain is normal or natural or has a purpose, can reduce our pain levels.[42] One piece of research identified two states of mind that women might experience during labour, which they called 'mindful acceptance' and 'distracted and distraught', with the latter consistently linked to higher levels of pain. Many different studies link the continuous support of a midwife the woman knows and trusts – so-called 'relationship-based care' – as a key factor in women's ability to cope.[43] And a study into how pain and pain relief impacts on 'childbirth satisfaction' ended by concluding that, in fact, pain didn't matter to women nearly as much as the attitudes of her caregivers, and being involved in decision-making. None of this is to minimise pain in labour or its importance, nor is it to suggest that women should give birth without any pain relief, in particular those who feel they both need it and want it, or who are placed in environments or settings where they do not receive the support they need to feel able to cope. It is slightly a chicken-and-egg situation, though, because if we keep telling women that labour is an agony that barely anyone can cope with, as well as pretending not to notice that we have built a birth system that's much more focused on the needs of the care provider than those of women, then women are going to keep needing pain relief and the system will never change.

When I gave birth myself, I noticed something that nobody had ever said to me, which was that labour is not painful all the way through. It's only the contractions that are painful (although some people prefer to call them surges or waves to help foster a more positive mindset). And the contractions are spread out, with time in between, in which you feel . . . normal? I'm not sure I'd call it that, because the cocktail of hormones you're producing can make you feel quite . . . trippy. Everything starts to take on a kind of starry, twinkly glow – and that's not just because of the tealights. When I wrote *The Positive Birth Book*, I decided to do the maths for an 'average' labour, and work out how much time you are actually in pain, versus how much time you spend in between contractions, with surprising results. What I discovered (and even I was surprised by this) is that the average labour is 77 per cent pain-free. With the help of several midwives, here's how I did the maths:

The average first stage of labour lasts about eight hours. I'm going to talk averages here for the purpose of our mental arithmetic, and of course, just as people can vary, so can these numbers. Bear with me, this is going somewhere – honest.

So. It's an eight-hour first stage. That's the bit when your cervix is dilating. For the first hour, you might have a contraction every twenty minutes. That's the bit that hurts. These contractions might last on average sixty seconds. So that's three in the first hour, lasting a minute each. That's three minutes of contractions. In hour two, they might come every ten minutes. So that's six contractions in the second hour of labour. By hour three, they might be coming 'two in ten' – that's two every ten minutes. So that's twelve contractions in hour three. For the next five hours of labour, things might really ramp up, so you are having 'three in ten'. That gives you a total of eighteen an hour, which in five hours adds up to ninety contractions.

So. In your eight-hour first stage, that's a total of 111 minutes of contractions. That's only 23 per cent of your time spent having contractions. The rest of the time, the other 369 minutes, the other 77 per cent, is entirely pain-free!

And the news gets better. Not every second of the sixty-second contraction is horribly painful. Most women only find the 'peak' of the contraction really tough, and that lasts about twenty seconds. Of your eight-hour first stage, only thirty-seven minutes will be spent at the peak of contractions. That's just 7.7 per cent.

So. That's 7.7 per cent of labour time that really, really hurts, and 15.3 per cent is moving towards or away from the peak of the contraction. And 77 per cent of labour that is pain-free.

To pre-empt the outcry that these calculations might elicit, I also did the maths for the 'nightmare labour from hell', the kind the man at the pub who keeps asking you about your pain-relief plans will tell you about – 'straight off the blocks at top speed and with four contractions every ten minutes for thirty-six hours', as I put it. And the numbers were still surprisingly positive.

If you're having a one-minute contraction, four times every ten minutes, for thirty-six hours, that's 864 minutes spent in pain, out of 2,160 minutes of labour – 40 per cent contractions; 60 per cent pain-free.

The extra-tough peak of contractions will take up only around 13 per cent of your labour. Heading up to the peak and back down again will take up 27 per cent of your time. The other 60 per cent of your time – you are not in pain.

This is the kind of reframe that the labour conversation needs. I like it, too, because it's not denying that the pain exists, or that some of the pain is flipping horrendous (I've had three babies, and it is). It's simply looking at it from a new angle and saying, 'This is what you've got to endure, and you can do it.' Like the woman in the Indian restaurant, it's saying, 'It's not that bad.' This doesn't change what labour is actually like, but it does change the mindset of pregnant women from, 'I don't know if I'll be able to cope with this,' to, 'I think I'm strong enough.' And as any marathon runner or mountaineer or elite sportsperson will tell you, mindset is everything. We don't say to these people, 'What if you die?' or, 'You know how much this is going to hurt, don't you?' even though people do die running marathons and most physical challenges involve moments of excruciating pain. And we know that after the race is won or the peak is conquered, elite athletes often feel superhuman. So we say: 'You've got this, you are up to this challenge.' Is it so hard to say this to the pregnant woman in the supermarket queue?

The problem is, this can make the woman in the supermarket queue feel judged, as if you are telling her that there is a right way and a wrong way to give birth, and that if she chooses a medicated birth in hospital, she's somehow failing. It would be great if we could move to a place of having these conversations without this happening, primarily by women all agreeing an absolute embargo on the idea that other women, even though they seem well meaning, actually have a hidden agenda to shame and criticise. It would also help if the concept of 'freedom of choice' was unpicked a bit more. All of us, even though we think we are free, often make choices that are a direct result of our cultural wallpaper, and in which we are limited by the situations we find ourselves in, and the information we are working with. In the 1920s, as women fought for equal voting rights with men, they also fought for another right: to a powerful labour drug known as 'twilight sleep'. At the time, childbirth was horrendous, with women facing either home birth attended by doctors extremely keen to use their forceps (of course, without local or regional anaesthetic), or dirty, crowded 'lying-in' hospitals, where death was at epidemic proportions due to doctors giving women sepsis with their unwashed hands. Twilight sleep – a mix of morphine and the powerful narcotic and amnesiac scopolamine – became part of the feminist discourse about women's rights and autonomy, and offered a seemingly perfect way for women to absent themselves from birth completely by placing them in an alternate state of consciousness. However, rather than being 'in control' as they imagined, the women who took this drug were instead wild and distressed, often having to be placed in padded beds, tied down or even straitjacketed. Afterwards, they would remember nothing, often not even believing they had given birth, and with friction burns, disassociation, flashbacks and an inability to bond with the baby they did not recognise. Of course, hospital birth with an epidural in 2026 is hopefully not comparable to these brutal births 100 years ago; however, what women then and now *do* have in common is that they have been told that the empowered thing to do is to numb themselves against an absolutely horrendous experience, rather than rebel full-scale against those who have denigrated childbirth into something that women wish so fervently to escape. They have been convinced that this is just 'how birth is'; it is the curse of their female biology, and there is no better way.

There is a better way. Women's bodies are not failing them; they are being failed by a system that does not listen to them and does not centre their needs, and, in the process, are deprived of a life-changing experience that puts them directly in touch with their unparalleled strength. We have to ask: is this deliberate? Is there something about childbirth that is so extraordinarily, mind-bendingly, essentially powerful that our patriarchal world has contrived to transform it instead into the ultimate proof of female inadequacy? So much so that the narrative has been changed at every level, even claiming that the power to create the world itself is held by a male God. On the surface, we may have bought into this myth, but as we journey through life in the female body, and experience each revolution of the matriflux, we must surely begin to have doubts. The female power each of us holds is older and stronger than the dominant narrative; we may hear it as a small yet persistent voice, or feel it as an intermittent surge of energy, in the twinge of ovulation, the throb of a menstrual cramp, the pulse of a multiple orgasm or the white heat of a labour contraction. There it is, every time we bleed but don't die, like the strongest of warriors. It's there and we feel it again and again: this power within.

Chapter 5

Mother Myths

"I have given up my membership of the world I used to live in."

RACHEL CUSK, *A Life's Work: On Becoming a Mother*

In the early years of my own experience of mothering – around 2012 – some curious images began to do the rounds on Facebook, of photographic baby portraits from the mid-nineteenth century. In the black-and-white pictures, something very strange is happening: the baby is seated on a person's lap, but this person is draped in a variety of fabrics – imagine someone with a tablecloth over their head, and you'll get the idea. There are hundreds of these portraits in existence, so much so that they've been archived, exhibited, made into a book and even given a name – they are 'The Hidden Mother' photos.[1] Apparently it was difficult to get babies to keep still for the long exposure times required for early photography, hence the need for a lap and a firm pair of hands, all clumsily disguised by an old pair of curtains. Another theory is that, because infant mortality was so high in these times and parents would often have posthumous pictures taken of their babies, parents actually wanted the hidden mother to look obvious, because her presence under the sheet signified that this particular baby was thankfully still alive and wriggling. Whatever the reasoning, it's hard to understand why the mother could not simply be visible in the photo. At the same time, her very obvious attempt to blend into the background feels eerily relatable. So needed, so vital – both for the emotional security of the child and the practicality of the photograph – and yet still obliged to conceal herself, not just from the photographer and contemporary viewers of the portrait, but from those who, like me, would look at the picture a hundred years later and only be able to see the great efforts she had made to erase herself, rather than her eyes or face.

When I had my first baby, I was convinced it would not change me in the slightest. I was 32, and had spent my twenties walking across the bridges of various big-city rivers with a cigarette in my hand and only a very loose plan, which felt fine. I liked the feeling of my own set of keys in my pocket; the spontaneity of a new flat, a new lover, or driving my clapped-out car to a new city in the days before satnav, when getting lost was always going to be part of the experience. When pregnant, I realised mothers and babies were largely absent from my social world, but somehow I thought that things would be different for me, a sort of maternity version of being 'not like other girls', perhaps. I didn't like shopping for baby stuff, preferring my best friend's advice that 'all you need is a pair of tits and a sling'. This sounded like freedom. But then, something surprising happened: I gave birth to an actual baby. As strange as it sounds, I don't think I anticipated this until the moment she was placed in my arms, her head cone-shaped from a difficult delivery, like a little alien. To me she was perfect; I felt as if I had always known her. Not only did I like being with her, but as a therapist who had specialised in attachment, I knew my presence had a value. I didn't particularly want to leave her with someone else, and even if I did, breastfeeding made this more complex. But ideas of going places with her in tow began to melt away as the reality sank in that this was a real person with huge needs that didn't have anything to do with city breaks, parties or long car journeys. Self-employed, I didn't have a high-flying job to return to, so I did a bit here and a bit there, but if anyone asked, I was 'mostly just a mum'. A second baby compounded this, and by the time I was looking at 'The Hidden Mother' photographs online in the early 2010s, I was living rurally and remotely with a 4-year-old and a 2-year-old and struggling to leave the house, not because I didn't want to, but because leaving the house with children of that age seemed to me an almost impossible task. Tired, overwhelmed and isolated, I heard the hidden mothers speak to me from beneath their slightly comical disguises: '*We see you.*' Like them, I had disappeared. Like them, I had played an active part in my disappearance, willingly placing the sheet over my own head.

This is just one version of my early-motherhood experience. I could tell you about it from a multitude of angles. I could make it sound idyllic, curating it like an exhibition and presenting you with blackberry-stained fingers, sandy toes, sunflowers, cupcakes, little hands in mine. Or I could make it sound like it ruined my life; the loneliness, the drudgery, the clear sense that I had become invisible. In truth, it was all of these things. Becoming a mother both broke me and made me again in a different shape. Childbirth took me across a threshold and there was no way back to the life I had had, or even to the person I had been. And I miss that person, just like I sometimes miss myself age 9 and wish I could spend a morning with my dad fixing up a rope and basket to hike essential items up to my treehouse, such as my latest library book or my guinea pig. But I am 51, and my dad is dead, and I can't be a child again, just as I can't be childless again. And if I could, I wouldn't want to be, because every day with my kids feels like the best bit of life, and my biggest fear is the inevitable future when the wheel cranks forward again into the next phase and they are no longer under my roof. Motherhood is wave after agonising wave of realisation about time, mortality and the fragility of existence, with added sandwich-making.

If you are a mother, perhaps you relate. Maybe you've also wished time away with your kids and then been devastated to find your wish came true: the time was gone. Maybe you also feel like you've spent every day since the birth of your first child trying frantically to adapt to each new phase of parenting and then, just as you begin to feel mildly confident – *bam!* – you are blindsided by a new, completely alien phase you have no knowledge or experience of. And this constant cycle of 'resentment – adaptation – mourning' is familiar, isn't it, because it's part of the wider fabric of our lives as women, too. It is the matriflux. Puberty, menstruation, pregnancy, breastfeeding, menopause; it seems like being a woman is a lifetime of consistently having to get to grips with change, and at the same time grieve the loss of a previous phase which, while it was actually happening, we often couldn't wait to be over. Motherhood is the microcosm of this macrocosm; our relationship with it a reflection of our relationship with womanhood itself. But could we potentially transform this relationship if we removed one element from the cycle – the resentment? Because, in my experience, this resentment often has its roots in feeling sidelined, unnoticed, invisible, undervalued. Perhaps, as well as reassessing our relationship with and respect for the female body, we also need to make peace with 'the mother': with our own mothers, with the mothers in our culture (so often invisible or unheard), with our role as mother (if we are one or wish to be one), with our internalised 'mother' archetype (whether or not we ever physically birth children, we still hold within us the capacity to 'mother', whether this is other people's children, or passion projects such as books, organisations, charities or businesses) and with the planet, Mother Earth herself. Doing so does not have to involve idolising the role of mother and insisting it's something all women should do and enjoy every minute of. It's more about a cultural shift, a transformation of how we see and treat those who do choose to be mothers, so that women on this path feel honoured and respected, rather than, as they so often report, cast aside and isolated.

What Is a Mother?

Mother is a word with global resonance. In many languages, it has a similar sound – *madre* (Spanish), *mutter* (German), *matka* (Polish), *mor* (Danish, Swedish, Norweigan), *mitera* (Greek). For many babies, the diminutive 'mama' is the first word (Swahili, Indonesian, Polish, Russian, German, Slovak, Mandarin, English), or 'mamma' (Italy, Iceland, Latvia, Sweden), partly because of the ease of repetitive combinations of consonant and vowel, partly because of the lip-smacking 'mmm' discovered at the breast, partly because of the motivational power of hunger.[2] For at least some of us, it will be our last word, too, or our last sight: hospice nurses report that in their dying moments, people will call out for or even see visions of their mother.[3] We all have our own personal, complex sense of what 'mother' means, and what the experience of being 'mothered' was like for us, even if we are not female or are not mothers ourselves. In recent times, just as the definition of 'woman' has been called into question, the word 'mother' has also been debated. Both the High Court in the UK and the European Court of Human Rights have said no to trans parents who wish to redefine 'mother'. In two cases, trans men who have given birth (trans men are biologically female but identify as men) have asked to be named as 'father' on their child's birth certificate, and in another case, a trans woman (who is biologically male and fathered the child) has asked to be named as 'mother'.[4] The courts have so far said no, asserting that, legally at least, a person who carries and gives birth to a baby is a mother. This is true even in the case of surrogacy, where, in the UK at least, the birth mother will be named on the birth certificate and new parents will have to apply after the birth for a parental order or adoption. In other parts of the world where surrogacy is commercialised (for example, Greece or some US states), surrogate mothers are not named on the birth certificate and become demoted to 'gestational carriers', whether or not they have contributed genetically to the child. No matter what the law says, though, many adopted people will feel an inexplicable pull to discover the woman who carried them, and many born from a donor egg will likewise wish to find out more, even if they have an adoptive mother or parent they love completely. Biology brings its own connection, and mother means something – beyond bodies, beyond law, beyond words.

The deep physical and spiritual connection between mother and child is often treated with disregard in a patriarchal world. Women's creative and life-giving power is diminished, dismissed or written out of the story and replaced by male gods and warriors. Treated merely as vessels and dehumanised by terms such as 'gestational carriers', 'cervix havers', and 'bodies with vaginas', we are broken down into parts, which can then more easily be commercialised. What we own can be rented and sold: a 'uterus owner' can therefore monetise this body part, and those who purchase its services can disassociate the organ from the whole person, facilitated by the language. This can be seen vividly in news stories of a Western couple's 'struggle' to collect their surrogate's baby from Ukraine, in which all of the focus is on the emotional journey of the adoptive parents, and not on the birth mother or 'carrier', who, in spite of being postpartum and left behind in a war zone, is often neither named nor mentioned.[5] Prior to the Russian invasion, the Covid-19 pandemic prevented many Westerners from collecting their babies from Ukraine: in May 2020, the *New York Times* reported that 'at least 100 babies are stranded already and that as many as 1,000 may be born before Ukraine's travel ban for foreigners is lifted', again, with no mention of the surrogates or their particular plight.[6] Currenty, the global surrogacy industry is growing rapidly, with some projecting it to grow sixfold in value in the next decade to 130 billion dollars.[7] In the UK, fifty children a year were born through surrogacy to British parents in 2008, but that number is now closer to 500.[8] And whilst UK laws maintain that surrogacy must be altruistic, surrogates can now claim expenses of around fifteen thousand to twenty thousand pounds, paid monthly like a salary, making it a draw for women on a low income. UK law also doesn't stop would-be parents heading abroad where laws are less restrictive to find babies, most often to lower income countries, again raising the possibility of exploitation. In October 2025, the UN Special Rapporteur on Violence Against Women and Girls, Reem Al Salem, presented a report calling for all UN member states to abolish surrogacy, which many, including the organisation Surrogacy Concern, object to on the grounds that it 'removes babies from their mothers at birth, exploits women's poverty, is profoundly unethical and makes a tradeable commodity of children and women's reproductive abilities'.[9]

The human complications inflicted on the surrogacy industry by legislation, war, pandemic or simply women having opinions about when or where they give birth – or, worse still, changing their minds and feeling unable to hand over their newborns – could be a thing of the past if 'ectogenesis' or 'artificial wombs' become reality – and they've already been trialled in sheep.[10] If this seems dystopian, wait until you hear about 'whole-body gestational donation', which is, according to the academics who have proposed it, 'a novel suggestion for circumventing the moral problems of gestational surrogacy', in which 'female patients in a persistent vegetative state who had given prior written consent, could function as surrogates'.[11] Arguably, neither this nor ectogenesis nor even commercial surrogacy would be given the green light in a world that values and honours women, the mother and the mother–infant bond.

Only Connect

For now at least, most human babies will be born to a living, breathing woman whose intention is to raise them as her own. Shining a spotlight on the ways in which the majority of these women cross the threshold into motherhood gives us further information about how the female body is understood or valued. In the moment of birth and the hours that directly follow, the universe presents us with an intense series of opportunities to celebrate and elevate women's power, and for women to feel this power within themselves in ways that will reverberate through them for a lifetime and perhaps further, through generations. These opportunities are so often missed, replaced instead with a destructive power grab that underpins the myth of female inadequacy and plays out like a Shakespearian tragedy. On her back, surrounded by professionals telling her what to do, the woman delivers her baby to the waiting hands of strangers, often unaware that she could instead be upright, instinctive and the first person to touch her newborn, or even 'catch it' herself as it emerges from her own body. An atmosphere of panic pervades in which the woman is passive and her attendants active, the baby removed with urgency and, as one mother put it to me, 'held aloft like a hunting trophy'. An artist could do worse than capture this moment and use it as an allegory for the relationship of the patriarchy to female power. The ultimate symbolic act centres around the umbilical cord, the long conduit that runs between baby and placenta and supplies the baby with nutrient-rich, oxygenated blood throughout pregnancy.

At the moment of birth, as much as a third of the baby's blood volume is still in the placenta, and the cord continues to visibly pulsate as it delivers this source of oxygen, stem cells, red blood cells and iron direct to the newborn. In spite of this, here, too, the need to lay claim, measure and meddle continues. There is no clinical reason whatsoever to cut the cord immediately, and the evidence is now clear that professionals should practice 'optimal cord clamping', and wait at least a minute,[12] probably several minutes, before clamping and cutting.[13] Historically, it's thought that immediate clamping may have become standard in American hospital births in the early twentieth century, due to the introduction of various narcotics for pain relief that were having a visible impact on the baby.[14] The practice then became widespread in the Western world, and for reasons that no medical professional can rationally explain, even if the mother has not had any drugs during labour, the visible symbol of connection between woman and baby has been repeatedly severed as a matter of urgency, sometimes even before the baby takes its first breath. The baby may then be removed from the mother, even taken out of her sight, to be wiped, weighed, wrapped in blankets, measured or in some cases given a bath. Again, the use of pain relief such as chloroform is thought to have been the origin of this practice, with women rendered unable to care for their newborns while they recovered from heavy sedation. Added to this, the invention of the incubator, originally for premature babies, started to become standard for all newborns in hospital, where they were felt to be safer from infection and generally optimised for health, away from their mothers and instead under the watchful eye of nurses. By the Sixties and Seventies, ideas about bonding and attachment, previously not even considered, had started to affect policy, but certainly when I was born in England in 1975, I was taken away for the first night of my life and fed formula by nurses, and even today, in some parts of the world, separation remains standard practice.

Although many changes have been made, the legacy of the past 100 years of Western maternity care lingers, and becomes most apparent in the frenzied activity that often unfolds around the moments just after birth. In spite of a few decades of evidence into the umbilical cord, for example, the urge to sever the mother–infant connection seems overpowering, so much so that you can regularly find headlines of 'quick-thinking dads', caught out by a swift birth at home or in transit, and told by 999 call handlers to tie off the cord with a shoelace. The introduction of something as dirty as a shoelace – or even, in at least two news stories from 2022, the elastic from a Covid face mask[15,16] – into the proximity of a newborn is clearly not thought to be as risky as leaving the mother-baby connection in place, even though many cultures outside of the medicalised

West – and all other mammals – take a more relaxed approach, with chimps even carrying both cord and placenta around after the birth until the cord dries up and falls off naturally a few days later. Humans can do this, too, and some do, in a practice called 'Lotus birth', in which the placenta is packed in salt and herbs and the cord is left to detach in its own time. When I asked one mother what her reasoning was for choosing a lotus birth, I somehow expected her to claim health benefits. Instead, she replied simply, 'It's symbolic. The separation is not forced, it is allowed to happen naturally and in its own time.' This approach is shocking to some, highly counter-cultural, and sets the tone for a similar style of parenting, in which the attachment between mother, primary caregivers and child is nourished via practices like co-sleeping (sleeping with your baby in close proximity) and babywearing (carrying your baby in a sling) that Western parents only a few decades ago would have found unthinkable. Those who practise this kind of 'attachment parenting', however, are trying to break with the relatively short 'tradition' of prams and nurseries and distance. They are trying to get back to something – something older.

Lotus birth is symbolic of respect for both women's creative power and the mother–infant connection, and conversely, immediate cord-cutting is symbolic of our collective disregard and disrespect for it. But even if you don't buy this idea that there's an unconscious motivation deep in every health professional as they wield the clamp and scissors, there is plenty of evidence of the physical benefits of, as some campaigning midwives call it, 'waiting for white' – and not cutting the cord until the 'placental transfusion' of blood is complete. Research shows that waiting for just three minutes can have a wide range of benefits; for example, preventing iron deficiency in infants,[17] improved fine motor skills at the age of 4[18] and even, in premature babies, reducing mortality.[19] Now that the evidence is mounting for waiting, however, the clock is yet again watched, as researchers and clinicians debate the precise number of minutes to wait before making the cut, when in fact research has shown that this can vary depending on a variety of factors, including how the baby is breathing or if they are crying.[20] Others propose that the baby should be held lower than the placenta in order to allow the blood to better transfuse – which of course means that the doctor, not the mother, is cradling the newborn.[21] Always the urge to 'do something', always the urge to intervene.

And always the urge to commercialise. One group who are very much aware of the health-giving properties of 'cord blood' are those companies who offer the service of 'cord blood banking'. 'Your baby's umbilical cord could change their life,' they tell their potential customers, adding that it is 'the richest source of stem cells they will ever have'. For several thousand pounds, plus an annual fee, such companies will collect and bank the 'cord blood', storing it on the premise that it might be helpful in future if a) your child gets sick, and b) they become unwell with something that their personal cord blood can help with. At the moment, the chances of this are extremely small, thought to be as low as 1 in 200,000 during their lifetime.[22] Currently, many of the diseases that can be treated with cord blood transplants are not suited to the patient's own cells, which may themselves contain the same problematic mutations or precursor cells that are causing the disease in the first place.[23] Many parents are sold the idea that future treatments 'might' be developed in which their child's banked cells would become life-saving. But although some companies claim to use technology that allows 'delayed cord clamping', the elephant in the room is that the 'cord blood' that they say has such huge potential benefits is not really 'cord blood' at all – it's the baby's blood. Somehow we have arrived at a place where it holds more value in a plastic bag in a remote freezer than it does in the human body for which it was intended: this again speaks to our collective distrust of the maternal body and how it can be leveraged for financial gain.

A baby whose cord is immediately cut and who is taken away to be examined and measured will not just miss out on their full blood volume, they will also be deprived of another mammalian staple – immediate skin-to-skin contact with their mother. This instinctive desire that both women and their babies share, for the baby to be lifted, naked, up onto the mother's chest, has been and remains a part of human birth in all cultures beyond the West, and in all of human history.[24] That is, until very recently, with the separation of babies from their mothers then becoming routine for much of the twentieth century, and continuing in some settings even today. Most women will feel instinctively that they want to hold their baby close in this way, and babies appear to feel the same: if they are removed from skin-to-skin in the time immediately after birth they will make a distinct distress call, and mothers who hear this cry will strain to see their babies, ask after them and ask to be given them back. If the baby stays close, they will soon notice the nipple, which has darkened in pregnancy, and now changes shape, with the areola expanding and the Montgomery glands enlarging and releasing an odour (these are the little raised bumps we all have on our nipples). This odour is the odour of home, of mother, to which every human has their own lifelong relationship: in utero, the amniotic fluid that we drink is flavoured by the food our mothers eat and this influences the development of the olfactory bulb, the part of our brain involved in our sense of smell. The aroma of the Montgomery glands is similar; as a newborn we then touch the nipple and make hand-to-mouth movements, recognising the taste and feeling the urge to suck, where again we will find the familiar taste of home in our mother's milk. Through our childhoods, the flavours of the family table will usually continue to surround us, and no matter how far we travel as adults, we will always have a relationship to those familiar flavours, sometimes calling them 'comfort food'. In old age, many of us rekindle a fondness for these foods of childhood, and the connection they hold, all the way back to the breast, to the womb and to 'mother', our first home.

During skin-to-skin, the baby will also recognise the mother's voice (and often the voice of her partner, too), and this will stimulate them to look for the face and make eye-to-eye contact, a significant moment of bonding, which many people find astonishing when they see it captured by cameras and displayed on social media. So many of us alive today will have been deprived of this moment, either as babies or new parents, in which newborns quietly meet the eyes of their mothers and others around them with a clear and knowing gaze.

Left undisturbed to simply drink each other in, mother and baby are free to explore each other's faces, while all the time, the mother's chest is helping to keep the baby's temperature regulated, increasing if the baby is colder and decreasing if the baby is warmer. Studies have also shown that the baby's heart rate, breathing rate, blood pressure and glucose levels are kept more stable by skin-to-skin contact, and that the newborn microbiome is also being colonised – this is the diverse range of bacteria that live on the skin and inside the body of all humans – now known to play an important role in our health.[25] And the link between uninterrupted skin-to-skin and breastfeeding is also well documented – increasing levels of oxytocin and prolactin, both of which are involved in milk production, and making it more likely that breastfeeding will get off to a good start and continue for longer, too.[26]

Programmes such as the Baby-friendly Hospital Initiative from the World Health Organization (WHO) and UNICEF, along with grassroots activism, have meant that, in recent years, some respect has been restored to the post-birth mother–infant connection. However, this has been met with resistance at times. Midwife Jenny Clarke campaigned for skin-to-skin after caesarean in the mid-2010s, initially by repeatedly writing it on the operating-theatre whiteboard.[27] When it kept being rubbed off, she got fed up and wrote it in fifteen-inch-high letters on the wall, angering some, but gaining her the nickname #BanksyMidwife on Twitter (now X) and eventually bringing about a change in practice. Another midwife, Amanda Burleigh, campaigned for optimal cord clamping for fifteen years and eventually left the profession, feeling she was bullied for her persistence. Even the Baby Friendly Initiative itself has come under fire from lobby groups like the Infant Feeding Alliance and the Fed Is Best Foundation, who protest that evidence-based practices such as skin-to-skin guilt-trip new mothers and may even put babies in danger.[28,29] Initiatives that enhance mother-baby attachment are, to employ an overused word, triggering: it can be deeply painful to see a baby being held close, soothed and prioritised if that experience was disrupted or absent for you, even if you hold no conscious memories of it. Early attachment happens when we are preverbal, and as such it can manifest itself in our expectations, beliefs, feelings and reactions; since so many of us share this collective pain, it can cease to be personal and wind up shaping culture and policy. In our grief we may build and promote systems that ignore the needs of babies and, conversely, have visceral reactions to practices that centre baby's needs in a way that ours were not personally centred. A possible way forward would be to acknowledge and tend to our own mother wounds before our own views about mothering become shaped by unacknowledged loss.

Women still feel the need to write into their birth plans that they wish to have an uninterrupted first hour after birth – a time that in *The Positive Birth Book* I called the 'power hour' – and some of them will report that they still experienced what they felt was unnecessary interference or a rushed atmosphere around this time, in spite of their requests. This will be explained as 'everyone doing their best', which of course is usually true, but it also speaks to something deeper: our inability to trust women; our anxiety around the female body in powerful action; our lack of regard for the mother; our discomfort with the mother–infant connection; and, perhaps above all else, our casting aside of the 'motherbody' as soon as its reproductive work is done. At some level, women carry all of this forward into the phase that follows.

Getting Your Body Back

In pregnancy, you get miraculously big, but then you must get small again. If tabloid newspapers and magazines are to be believed, the goal of early motherhood is to try to erase any evidence that you have just had a baby, as fast as you possibly can. The ultimate achievement is to 'get your body back', and to be seen on the red carpet looking exactly as you did a year ago, with no baby in sight, either. Celebrity mums who use social media posts to share their bodies fall into the usual damned if you do, damned if you don't trap, with those whose bodies look toned and 'just the same as before' being praised and then in the same breath slammed for shaming women, and those who have more relatable postnatal curves being held up as role models one minute and viciously attacked in the comments section the next. Six months after giving birth to her second child, tennis star Serena Williams posted on Instagram in February 2024 about the importance of 'self-love', writing: 'Right now I love that my body is not picture perfect'[30]; just a few months later she sparked outrage by admitting she'd lost 31 lb using a GLP-1 weight-loss drug; now she's gone a step further and is promoting the jabs in adverts shown during the 2026 Super Bowl. It's quite possible public scrutiny of her and her fellow celebrities' bodies nudged her desire to be slimmer – now that she's achieved this, here's just a small a flavour of the comment section I'm reading today on her Super Bowl ad[31]:

Never been a fan. She still looks chunky.

My eyes need bleaching and wire brushing. What has been seen, cannot be unseen.

Nobody needs or wants to see this. Her husband really has a thing for the ugly . . .

She's a big girl.

Looks like she has a ball in her lower stomach. It's not pretty.

And so on . . .

Women's feelings about the inadequacy of their postpartum bodies can dominate the first months or even years of motherhood.[32] Cultural messaging about conforming to beauty standards plays a part, but what is less discussed is the psychological aspect of how women feel about their own mothers and childhood, and what it is therefore like for them to embody this role, and be reminded of it each time they stand naked in front of a mirror and see unfamiliar stretch marks, places that sag, rolls and curves. They feel the conflict of having to work like they are not a mother, mother like they do not work, and sense the impossibility of having it all, of being all things to all people: worker, sexual partner, mum. The emotional load of having to 'be there' for the family – knowing where everything is located, what is in the fridge, who needs extra support and why, and what time all of the clubs and appointments are, can begin the day after a first baby is born and continue for decades, and it wears women down. Perhaps the aspiration of the woman on the red carpet is about shedding more than baby weight – it's about setting down the load of motherhood itself and feeling the lightness of freedom again. In reality, of course, that's impossible, so we keep our bodies covered up and, notoriously, stay out of family photos, because rather than looking red-carpet ready, we look . . . like a mum, and we don't want a record of that.

The active breast

Breastfeeding is an intense experience in which your body is not entirely your own, and, in the collective imagination, it's perhaps the ultimate symbol of maternity – think Leonardo da Vinci's '*Madonna Litta*', or all those serene breastfeeding statues you'll find in churches. It's also another female bodily superpower – not only can we sustain life in the womb, but we can then sustain it outside for months with our milk alone. However good it may seem on paper or in the carved marble version, the reality can be very different, an activity where our relationship to our bodies, and our confidence in them, is tested yet again. Researchers have even found that women's body image can impact on their desire to breastfeed at all and, if they start, the length of time they continue for.[33] Women worry that their bodies – already, in their eyes, negatively impacted by pregnancy and birth – will take a further hit if they breastfeed, although some are spurred on by the idea that it may help them lose weight. Body concerns are also focused around feeding in public, exposing flesh that they already dislike to a wider audience. For every female anxiety, a product exists – women can purchase a 'breastfeeding cover' that drapes over them, rather like a wearable fabric tent, and not a million miles off the perfect accessory for a Victorian 'Hidden Mothers' photoshoot. Their concerns are very real: researchers from Swansea and Cardiff universities in 2022 described a 'hostile environment' for breastfeeders, in which 'the attention of members of the public who observed breastfeeding was incorrectly focused on mothers as sexualised women, rather than as caregivers to infants who needed feeding'.[34] In spite of it being illegal in the UK to ask a mother to stop breastfeeding in public,[35] this happens frequently: in car parks,[36] supermarket checkouts,[37] and perhaps most frequently, in swimming pools where, in spite of the fact that the pool contains children in nappies, and adults who may or may not have throroughly washed their most intimate areas, the idea of a woman's nipple being momentarily exposed or even (God forbid) dripping breast milk into the chlorinated water seems to really disturb people.[38] Incidents of women being told to stop nursing in public are often followed by 'phone-in' debates on the radio along the lines of, 'Should it be allowed?' and even though the law clearly already says, 'It is allowed,' there are always people willing to say how they support breastfeeding – 'But . . .'[39] The irony is often noted, of course, that the breast is already everywhere, on billboards, magazines and the red carpet, too. It seems that, rather like the body in childbirth, we only object to the breast's exposure when it is active, independent and purposeful, but don't mind it so much when it's selling us chocolate or underwear: passive, there only to be looked at. Even breastfeeding itself is exploited: at the time of writing the top four search results for me on Facebook for 'breastfeeding' are soft porn videos of large-breasted women pretending to nurse plastic dolls.

In reality the breast is clever. It doesn't just squirt out milk when the baby sucks, although that would arguably be clever enough. For starters, the milk changes and adapts depending on the baby. At birth, you get colostrum, which some refer to as 'liquid gold', a thicker, yellower substance, packed with antibodies, antioxidants, vitamins and nutrients in much higher quantities than in breast milk. Breast milk 'comes in' around three days after the birth, although the content changes gradually, establishing itself at around fourteen days. Production of colostrum starts during pregnancy, stimulated by progesterone from the placenta, then, when progesterone levels drop after the birth, milk production is triggered. But this is not the only time that changes happen in the breast milk composition – it adapts continually. If the baby sucks for a short time, they get a more watery, thirst-quenching milk, known as foremilk. If they keep sucking, they get the hindmilk, which is richer and higher in calories. Breast milk also changes as the baby grows,[40] perfectly tailoring itself to their age and development, with premature babies' milk being specifically higher in fat, calories and protein,[41] whereas milk for older babies and toddlers becomes increasingly richer in immunoglobins, perhaps to help give their immunity a boost at a time when they are on the move and therefore in contact with more germs.[42] Milk is different in the day and night, with night-time milk containing nucleotides, said to stimulate GABA, a sleep-inducing neurotransmitter,[43] and evening milk containing tryptophan, a sleep-inducing amino acid, which helps the baby make the sleep hormone melatonin (not that this ever seemed to work on my babies, who broke my sleep – and nearly broke me – for years on end).[44] And it gets better – when a mother kisses her baby, she samples pathogens on their face, which then travel to her lymphatic system, causing antibodies to be created, which the baby then receives through the milk. It's also thought that there is a complex feedback loop between the baby's saliva and the mother's nipple – with 'backwash' from the nursing child travelling back into the nipple and informing the breast about the baby's health needs,[45] causing antibodies to increase if they have a virus, and also helping to regulate the mouth and gut microbiome.[46]

We are rarely told or taught the incredible science of women's bodies. Breast milk even differs depending on whether the baby is male or female: the researcher Katie Hinde has documented that, in several species of mammal, including humans, sons get milk that is higher in protein and fat than daughters, but that daughters get milk in higher quantities. If you find this hard to believe, ask a dairy farmer: in the US dairy industry, large-scale farmers will pay extra for sex-selected insemination for their cows' first pregnancy – because if their first calf is female they will have a significantly higher yield over the next two lactations.[47] Why and how do we make sex-specific milk? Like so much of female biology, there is much we don't yet understand, simply because it's not been given much attention. A study in bank voles, where researchers cross-fostered their offspring to create all-male and all-female litters, and gave some of the voles larger or smaller litters to feed than they had gestated, has concluded that there is a *postnatal mechanism* that means the voles still make more milk for females.[48] But what this postnatal mechanism is – how the breast knows the sex of the offspring – is yet to be discovered. Data from the dairy industry shows that there is also a *prenatal mechanism*, programming the mammary gland to the sex of the offspring, probably through the sex-specific hormones of the male or female foetus crossing into the mother's circulation via the placenta. Again, our knowledge is limited, as it is for the question of *why* human mothers would make different milk for male or female babies, although researchers speculate this is because males and females have very different growth patterns, with fattier milk for boys, who have a larger body size, and less fat and more calcium for girls, whose skeletons are faster growing.[49]

Got Milk?

What we do know is that mothers notice the lesser volumes of milk for their boy babies, and that this is potentially fuelling their anxiety that they are suffering from 'insufficient milk' – male babies are more likely to be supplemented with formula and weaned earlier, and their mothers are more likely to seek advice for low supply than women with female babies. If you've got this far in this book, it won't come as a surprise to you to find out that, as in so many other areas, mothers of babies of both sexes have some serious doubts about their breastfeeding abilities, and that one of the main reasons women who do want to breastfeed have for stopping is their concerns about inadequate supply.[50] But, unless there are clear, ongoing concerns about a baby's weight gain, how does a mother know that she is not making enough? It's possible that very often this is simply a perception, so much so that the phenomena has been given a name: PIM, or perceived insufficient milk.[51] Any discussion about breastfeeding and the reasons for deciding to stop (or not to start in the first place) can be emotive, so let's be clear, if you are reading this and stopped nursing due to supply concerns, or for any other reason, this is not a judgement of your choices. Instead, it's seeking to highlight the bigger cultural picture, in which the myth of female bodily inadequacy pays yet another visit to women and yet again whispers absolute falsehoods in their ear that they are not up to the job. Around 81 per cent of UK women initiate breastfeeding after birth, but the numbers then fall off a cliff, with exclusive breastfeeding at six weeks at 24 per cent, three months at 17 per cent, and six months at 1 per cent. Although we are often told that how women feed their babies is down to 'personal choice', we also know that eight out of ten UK women stop breastfeeding before they want to.[52] Eight out of ten. We don't know how many of them stop because of PIM, probably for the same reason that PIM exists in the first place – because it's very hard to see or measure how much breast milk a woman is making. Having breastfed three babies, I can remember just how powerfully this lack of concrete information affected not only me, but others around me – family, health professionals, well-meaning strangers – all of us struggling at times to collectively trust that my female body, and the milk it produced, was 'enough'.

As if often the case, there is money to be made from this particular body myth. Into this area of insecurity and doubt steps the formula industry, offering women clear certainty about the amount of milk their babies are drinking, with global profits of around 55 billion dollars a year. In the West, part of the lack of confidence in the breast's abilities comes from the intergenerational damage that has been done by formula marketing. Let's not forget that, circa 1960, families were being told that formula was not just a good replacement for breast milk, as they are now, but that it was vastly superior. My own dad, born in 1926 (he had me at 49), was somewhat baffled by my commitment to breastfeeding. 'Formula milk is better,' he told me, and he really did mean it. 'Something that's made by experts in a lab is bound to be an improvement on something made by a body!' When parents of his generation fed their babies a bottle in the Sixties and Seventies, it felt like a great advancement, but it simultaneously created a broken chain of wisdom, in which the traditional way mothers were helped and supported to breastfeed – by older women with personal experience – was removed from the culture. Questions like that of my dad ('What's wrong with formula?') or a lack of understanding of how breastfeeding works ('Are you feeding that baby again? You only just fed him!', 'Do you think she is waking at night because she is hungry?', etc.) all sow seeds of doubts in the fertile landscape of women's perceived inadequacy. Another legacy of formula feeding, the 'scheduled' feeds, encourages women to watch the clock rather than learn and respond to their baby's hunger cues, while other body myths – for example, that larger breasts make more milk, that leaking is a sign of good supply or that all women feel engorgement or a strong sensation as the milk flows at 'let-down' – can all contribute to a lack of conviction.[53] As always, there are highly dubious gadgets and apps that claim to solve the problem by measuring milk output: 'Know how much your baby is getting,' says one, promising to solve, once and for all, this tiresome female mystery and its bothersome requirement of body confidence. All of these worries can prompt women to supplement with a bottle, which in turn interferes with the supply–demand system of breastfeeding, and can, ironically, initiate genuine supply issues, leading to the need for additional formula. To reiterate, any woman who does not wish to breastfeed should not have to feel bad about that, but the reality is that many women end their breastfeeding journey feeling disappointed – 'I wanted to breastfeed, but I wasn't able' – and yet again have their emotions shut down by being told that it 'doesn't matter', and that 'fed is best'. Again, they feel they have 'failed', when in fact they have *been* failed by a highly unsupportive culture that ultimately prefers its breasts in porn and its milk from a cow. Again, women are deprived of an empowering physical experience and sold the lie that they were 'insufficient'. Again, women and their bodies are wrongly blamed. And again, money is made from the false story of female inadequacy.

Like the milk itself, the contribution of breastfeeding to society is not always visible or easy to measure. We can look at the time women spend doing it – conservative estimates suggest around 1,800 hours in a year of breastfeeding, which is not far off the hours that would be spent in a forty-hour-a-week full-time job – although, of course, breastfeeding has no weekend breaks or annual leave, and is spread out through nights as well as days.[54] But even if we use traditional surveys for 'time use', these don't tend to capture the complexity of mothers' lives, in which both breastfeeding and caring for other children may be performed simultaneously, as well as other tasks (as a case in point, I wrote many articles and large chunks of my first book while breastfeeding). Another way of measuring is to look at GDP, but Norway is the only country in the world that makes any attempt to count the economic contribution of breastfeeding. This global blind spot to women's impact is symptomatic of our patriarchal society's dismissal of women's power; as the WHO Council on the Economics of Health For All put it, 'Pregnancy, childbirth and lactation are at the centre of health for all, but since human reproduction is women's work, these activities do not count.' By not including human milk in GDP calculations, we can actually give a false impression of economic progress, explains Dr Karleen Gribble, infant feeding specialist and adjunct associate professor at Western Sydney University. 'The fact that breastfeeding is not counted in economic measurements means that when mothers are not supported to breastfeed and, as a result, infant formula sales increase, GDP also increases. The costs of reduced breastfeeding, including in terms of increased illness in infants and mothers, are overlooked, and the undermining of women and children's rights ignored.' Breastfeeding is about more than just milk – it is nurture, love, attachment and highly optimised nutrition with a lifelong health impact; as important to humans as hugs and time spent in nature, and equally difficult to quantify.

Like menstruation, pregnancy and even menopause, breastfeeding is at first glance a spanner in the works of gender equality. If we see it simply as an activity that 'holds women back' from the freedom, careers and status that men enjoy, then it is easy to arrive at the conclusion that formula milk really is 'liberation in a can', as those who market it have long claimed. Like childcare and mothering, breastfeeding is dismissed as care work, which is often regarded as demeaning and something that nobody should aspire to. But this is not how many women see it. In countries where policies have been introduced to encourage male and female partners to take equal and separate parental leave, women have often chosen to decline, partly because, in particular for those who breastfeed, this form of 'equality' is unworkable, and partly because many women (and I was one) actively enjoy this time with their infants. Supporting women to do this work has far-reaching benefits: paid maternity leave has a demonstrable positive impact on women's mental and physical health, even in the long term and particularly in those who are single and socioeconomically disadvantaged. Several studies have also shown maternity leave to be literally life-saving to babies: in one, each additional month of paid maternity leave was associated with 7.9 fewer infant deaths per 1,000 live births;

in another, infants of women who accessed unpaid maternity leave had almost half the risk of being hospitalised as compared to infants of mothers who did not access maternity leave. In another, babies whose mothers took maternity leave were 16 per cent less likely to die from congenital abnormalities or undefined causes (such as sudden infant death syndrome – SIDS) compared to infants of demographically similar women who did not take maternity leave.[55]

Shadow Boxing

In spite of such benefits, it is still a widely held and, for some, feminist view that true equality can only come from all care work being shared fifty-fifty between the sexes, and in an imagined future this may well look like a laboratory-grown baby who is fed formula by robots and possibly even raised by them, too, with all the messy inconvenience of female biology erased. For now, though, motherhood and the damage it can wreak on the ambitions, careers, lives and bodies of unsuspecting women in the prime of their lives remains a problem to be solved. For many, this brings an ambivalence towards motherhood, manifesting in current trends of having fewer children, having children much later or deciding not to have them at all.[56] Some women are now speaking openly about regretting having children, summarised by one mother who wrote in an article for *Today's Parent*, 'What I'm struggling with is that it feels like their amazing life comes at the expense of my own.'[57] Her account is extremely relatable – the isolation, the invisibility of her own needs, the exhaustion, the relentlessness, and the jealousy of the freedom of child-free friends to drop everything and travel or party. Because I write about pregnancy and birth in positive terms, people are sometimes surprised when I say I've had all those negative feelings and more in my eighteen years of parenting, and that I fully understand and support any woman who chooses to ditch motherhood completely and use her female creative energy in other ways. The ability to tolerate ambivalence, and acknowledge and express a complex range of emotions, in particular those that are contradictory, is extremely healthy. If we push down or disown thoughts and ideas that we perceive to be negative or unacceptable, we run the risk of creating what Carl Jung called the 'shadow', a dark place of unacknowledged feelings that we have to work hard to maintain do not belong to us. Shadows are particularly likely to be created in areas where there is a great deal of 'light', so it's unsurprising to find them around motherhood, which is so often glorified as a completely unrealistic state of perfection: the dainty crib, the nursery bunting, the pretty mother rocking her contented baby. Behind this glowing golden scene there's a dark shadow lurking, and into it goes the stench of an overflowing nappy bin, the exhaustion so powerful you lose the ability to make sentences, the regret, the isolation, the loss. I can remember wanting sleep so badly when my first child was a baby that while I was nursing her at 3 a.m., I wondered about deliberately getting myself run over, just lightly enough to break a couple of bones and get me a week of luscious respite in a hospital bed. These are the shadowy moments we are not supposed to mention.

'Heaven lies at the feet of your mother.'

PROPHET MUHAMMAD

Social media blasts some light in: memes tell us, 'The struggle is real,' or they show us other mums with their mess and chaos. But for every one of those, there's another where everything looks neat and idyllic. It's almost as if our inner battle between the light and dark of motherhood is playing out on social media in real time, as we collectively try to work through our feelings, the 'dream' versus the very challenging 'reality'. There is not a corresponding number of dads sharing their lives in this way; it is mums and only mums, and whether they show us fresh flowers on the empty worksurface or the overflowing laundry basket, the underlying need is the same: *See me. Appreciate me. Double tap. Value me.* Sometimes, the centre cannot hold, and the shadow side bursts through unexpectedly. The 'mumfluencer' Clemmie Hooper, known as @Mother_of_Daughters, had over 700,000 followers on her Instagram account, which showed a picture-perfect life of little twin girls with ringlets, an immaculate kitchen and an enviable wardrobe of trend-setting outfits. But Hooper had a shadow. Upset by online criticism, in 2019 she created a secret, fake account on *Tattle Life* – a dark, bitchy forum where people let loose all the hatred and scorn that looking at photos of a person's new marble worksurface can elicit. On *Tattle Life* (itself a shadow side of online influencer culture, and incidentally, run by a man using a female pseudonym), Hooper tellingly called herself 'Alice in Wanderlust' – which has a subversive, adventurous vibe in contrast to the homespun,

'Mother of Daughters' – and began to join in with discussions about herself.[58] To make her fake account seem more authentic, she wrote horrible things about her fellow influencers, some of whom were her friends. She was caught out and publicly shamed, and her Instagram, with all its followers, advertising deals and statement lighting, went dark overnight, never to return.[59] It's easy to see Hooper herself as flawed, and like most of us, she probably is. But there's a reason she fell so dramatically from grace, and it's probably more to do with the impossibility of carrying the weight of 700,000 other women's projections than any specific fault in her nature. Being on a pedestal is precarious, and finding yourself on that pedestal in a terrazzo-tiled shrine, dressed in matching family pyjamas and beatified as the patron saint of motherhood is only going to go one way.

Speaking Words of Wisdom

Turn a little corner in the grounds of my Catholic primary school and you found something surprising: behind a few bushes and trees and built into the right angle of the red-brick walls was a 'grotto'. Like a sort of large rockery, the grotto was built up with stones and plants into a pinnacle, at the top of which was a statue of Mary, whom Catholics call Our Lady. Robed in white, with a blue cloak and outstretched palms, she looked serenely downwards, and, in my memory at least, some of the little nooks and crannies in the rocks were filled with candles that glowed in red glass lanterns, amid the flowers. As a child, I found this place enchanting. Perhaps something meshed in my mind with another type of 'grotto' – the Father Christmas variety – but I definitely knew and expected that magic happened here. Although I wasn't Catholic myself, I was immersed in their faith, taught by nuns who told me that magic most certainly did happen, in their stories about miracles, healing waters and the apparitions of Mary to little girls like St Teresa and St Bernadette. Little girls just like me. Then there was the rosary, pretty beads that the nuns could purchase for you in a variety of colours – even glow-in-the-dark – and the 'medals of Our Lady' in vivid transparent blue. I wanted one of them so badly that I swapped my best bouncy ball for it. And sometimes in my lunch hour I would go to the school chapel alone – another place filled with images of Mary – stare hard at the wall and pray, pray, pray for her to appear. I don't think I had any illusions of grandeur or desire for fame. I just believed in the magic and wanted it to happen to me.

As an adult, I've wondered for a long time why Mary captured my imagination so powerfully as a child, and if maybe all it means is that I was a bit of a weird kid. It wasn't until relatively recently, when I started reading and learning about both the divine feminine and matriarchal cultures that it suddenly started to make sense. As Sharon Blackie puts it in *If Women Rose Rooted*, 'It wasn't that I wanted to replace a male god with a female god; it wasn't that I wanted to find a religion at all. I was simply looking for some sense that women might have worth.' Mary – who the Catholics are always very keen to stress is not 'worshipped' but rather 'venerated' – is, in all other ways, a goddess of sorts. It is thought that when Christianity was taking hold, followers of older religions and belief systems were used to more of a balance of masculine and feminine deities than the male-dominated idea that just one Father god offered. A goddess figure was needed to create a bridge between old and new ways, and the idea of a 'mother of God' worked perfectly. Mary, with her pagan associations of healing springs, the sea (she is known as *Stella Maris* or 'Star of the Sea') and the moon (as the Queen of Heaven), holds much in common with other, older female deities, such as: Kali, the Hindu 'mother of the universe'; Isis, the Egyptian life-giving mother and healer; the Irish goddess of fertility, spring and poetry, Brigid; and Demeter, the Roman harvest-mother goddess. Of particular importance at the time of early Christianity was Cybele, known as the Great Mother, or *Magna Mater.* Cybele held a cult-like status, originally in Asia Minor and then among the Greek and Roman empires, and is thought by some scholars to have been the model for Mary herself. The importance of the divine feminine to people goes back further still: hundreds of paleolithic 'Venus' figurines (as they are called by their modern discoverers) have been discovered across Europe. The scholar Max Dashú has argued that they should not be called 'Venus' but rather 'female icons' or 'ancestral mothers', because Venus is a Eurocentric term and 'projects a narrow presumption of "sex object" onto iconography that has a far broader range of meanings and ceremonial uses'.[60] The oldest of these female icons, the Venus of Hohle Fels, dates back to 40,000 years ago and is described as 'the oldest known depiction of a human'. But with her large, visible vulva and enormous breasts, she is not just human – she is female.

When you think about it, it makes complete sense that the ultimate creator would be female. It is women who can create life, growing it in their bodies and nurturing it from their breasts. If anything, it's hard to understand why people have ever been convinced that the complete opposite – as we see in the Bible, in which woman is born from a man's body – is true. The positioning of male-only deities as the source of life is now a part of most major world religions, and even if, like me, you have no religious faith, your life, education and sense of self will have been affected by this story being part of your cultural background. And of course the story is accompanied by the widespread idea that men are the ultimate authority, played out in the structure of our social worlds under patriarchy. This myth of superior male power is starkly challenged and upended by birth and breastfeeding – which may be in part why the little girl who was so enchanted by Mary went on to become deeply interested in women's power – or lack of it – in the birth room. Patriarchy must convince us not only that God is male but that 'power' is entirely about domination and rule, and so we are taught that the female body in childbirth is weak and vulnerable, and in school, we learn that our history consists of wars, conquests and colonisation. We are never taught that this is just one version of events (his story) and that there might be other stories (her story), and other ways for humans to coexist. We are never taught about matriarchy.

When people first hear about matriarchy, there is an assumption that it is simply female rule and domination instead of male – effectively the same system we already have but with women in charge. In fact, matriarchy is an entirely different system of living, based on 'motherly values' of nurture and care. As HAGIA, an academy dedicated to the study of matriarchal societies, explains, 'In matriarchies, mothering – which originates as a biological fact – is transformed into a cultural model.'[61] Socially, maternal values of unconditional love and support are adopted by everyone, not just mothers, and not just women, and people live in large kinship groups, with titles and status passed through the mother line, and goods evenly distributed by the matriarch or clan mother. Politically, matriarchies are organised as egalitarian, with decisions made democratically and by consensus. And spiritually, the entire ethos of the matriarchy is built on the notion of the divine feminine or goddess. The matriarchy is not a place of 'power over', but of 'power within'; communities that nurture and care for each other just as the mother cares for her child and the Earth itself nurtures and sustains human life. Matriarchies still exist around the world: the Hopi of North America or the Mosuo in China, for example, and scholars of matriarchy argue that it was the original way of life until around 5,000 years ago. But the very idea of matriarchy – rather like the idea of female deities – is controversial and oft-disputed, for the obvious reason that it is extremely challenging to the long-established status quo, which suits those in charge – men – nicely, thank you very much.

Like the buried paleolithic goddesses that continue to be unearthed, much of women's history and power remains covered up and hidden. New mothers perhaps reflect this when they feel isolated, cast aside and invisible, where they should be cherished, celebrated or 'worshipped'. Regardless of whether ideas about matriarchy and the divine feminine resonate with you, it can't be denied that our relationship with the Earth – who we think of as 'Mother' – is currently broken; she also feels cast aside rather than cherished. The mother in us feels this, too: hence a 'dad bod' may be sexy but a 'mum tum' is not; we must not be 'mumsy'; we must not dress 'like a mum'; we must not 'sound like our mothers' or (God forbid) our mothers-in-law. We are 'selfish mothers', 'bad mothers' and 'toxic mothers', or, if we're lucky, 'good enough mothers', subject to more scrutiny and judgement than fathers by about a hundred-fold. Our focus through patriarchy has been to denigrate the mother and then exploit her; to own her and to dominate her and to control her. We need to shift our energy away from this and towards matriarchal values of relationship, connection, nurture and a new kind of power, the kind that is not used to destroy or to rule over, but to create.

There's something else that's interesting about paleolithic goddesses as well. They may all look like 'mothers', but they're definitely not the red-carpet ready variety. They have curves, bulges, rounded bellies that sag and roll, breasts that hang like ripe fruit, nipples that point southwards, bottoms that are wide and sturdy. They are often said to be symbols of fertility, but in truth they look more like women who have already been there and done that, quite a few times. To me, it seems like the goddess with all her power and wisdom wasn't a young fertile mother at all, but a solid and reliable middle-aged woman.

Chapter 6
Menopause Myths

'At menarche a woman meets her power,
through bleeding she practises her power,
at menopause she becomes her power.'

NATIVE AMERICAN SAYING

Not long after my third and final baby stopped breastfeeding, I started to wake up bathed in sweat. I was in my early forties, and when I mentioned it in an online group, the answer quickly came: 'Oh, yeah. That's peri.' It took me a while to work out what they meant. Peri? Isn't that a type of cider made from pear juice? A spicy chicken sauce? You what now? The peri-*menopause*? You've got to be kidding, right? I've only just started to finally get some sleep after a decade of pregnancy, crying newborns and toddlers that want to gnaw on my nipples all night. I've literally had about two blissful months of getting into bed every evening and knowing I probably won't get woken up by anything until someone says, 'Mummy, I've done a poo,' in my ear at about 6 a.m. And now you're telling me I'm MENOPAUSAL?! IS THERE NO RESPITE FROM THIS WOMANHOOD BS??!!

And anyway, I thought, once I'd calmed down a bit, I'm only 43. I can't possibly be menopausal, peri or otherwise. I'm just not ready to think of myself in that way. Menopausal, to me, meant 'past it'. Life over, old, grey, saggy and, basically, not a hotty anymore, unless you count the night sweats. Several years later and, to be honest, I still don't know if it was 'peri', or if it was just my body adjusting to no longer breastfeeding, which – as I'd fed three babies back to back since my first was born in my early thirties – must have been quite a seismic hormonal transition in itself. The sweats stopped after a few months. Then, a couple of years after that, I went through eighteen months or so of feeling completely exhausted, aching all over, and my periods became very irregular. I started weight training and began to feel better. Then, my periods became more regular again, and then, after I had my first covid jab (and, although there have been some questions raised about the impact of this particular vaccination on the menstrual cycle, I will never know if this was a coincidence), they stopped suddenly and almost completely when I was 48. In the midst of this rollercoaster few years, I never really knew what was going on, and there didn't seem to be anyone who could reliably tell me. There is no accurate test for perimenopause. I'm a woman, and my body is a mystery, basically. Not just a mystery, either, but a mystery that is seemingly in an almost constant state of transformation: puberty – pregnancy – postpartum – breastfeeding – the intense and rapid changes of motherhood – perimenopause – menopause; a lifetime of the matriflux, in which the only thing that stays the same is change.

Menopause actually means the state you reach when you haven't had a period for a year, and on average this happens to women in their early fifties. When people talk about the menopause, they are usually describing perimenopause, the time leading up to menopause itself, which in the average woman lasts around four to six years, but can be shorter or longer – and in some cases can last up to ten years. During this time, fertility begins to slowly decline; ovulation may happen less regularly, progesterone drops and oestrogen levels spike and then ultimately fall. Why human females outlive their fertility for so many decades remains a mystery to science. Only two other species, the orca, or killer whale, and the pilot whale, continue to thrive once their capacity to reproduce has come to an end, but more on this later.

Although there's not a test to see if you are in perimenopause, a blood test will establish if you have reached menopause itself by measuring your level of follicule-stimulating hormone (FSH) – post-menopausal women have it in much higher levels than ever before in their life. This is because FSH (which is part of reproduction in both males and females) is released by the pituitary gland during the first half of the menstrual cycle to stimulate the ovaries to prepare an egg for ovulation. As this happens, in pre-menopausal women the dominant follicle will produce oestrogen as it grows, which, when it peaks, sends a signal to the brain to produce another hormone, luteinising hormone (LH), which in turn, triggers the release of the egg. Without oestrogen – much less of which is produced during perimenopause and after menopause – ovulation doesn't happen, which means that the second half of this hormonal 'loop' doesn't happen either. Instead of FSH being inhibited, the levels of this hormone just keep rising – high enough to signal in a blood test that you're officially in menopause, and as much as twenty times higher than they were when you were having a menstrual cycle. By the time they are this high, though, you're likely to know you're in menopause anyway, because your periods will probably have completely stopped: no ovulation = no monthly period.

To put menopausal levels of FSH into perspective, a positive result for menopause is usually considered to be anything over 30 mIU/mL. In a pre-pubescent girl levels are around 0 to 4, during puberty between 0.3 and 10, and post-puberty while still cycling, between 4.7 and 21.5 (with the highest levels at ovulation). After menopause, 30 mIU/mL is the minimum level to indicate you're no longer ovulating, but FSH levels can be much, much higher, even up to and above 100. When I first read about this, I felt curious: does this extremely high level of FSH have an impact on us, or maybe even a purpose? I was unable to find an answer: all descriptions of high FSH relate to negative experiences such as lack of sleep and unwanted weight gain. It seems only to be understood as a hormone of reproduction, and whether or not it plays a positive or important role in the body appears never to have been explored. Perhaps there is an assumption that the high post-menopausal levels are yet another misfire of the female body, for which thankfully medical science can compensate. This same pathologising lens is used to examine perimenopause itself, which is almost always described as a set of 'symptoms': hot flushes, mood changes, night sweats, trouble sleeping, palpitations, weight gain, headaches and migraines, reduced sex drive, muscle aches and joint pain, vaginal dryness and recurring UTIs.[1] The whole package sounds vastly unpleasant, but the good news is, it's apparently pretty much avoidable, thanks to the medication known as HRT.

From Mares to Maga

Hormone replacement therapy, or HRT, has a chequered past. In the late 1920s, a scientist called Edward Adelbert Doisy was the first to isolate the hormone oestrogen while studying the urine and follicular fluid of pigs.[2] By the 1930s, oestrogen was already being marketed as a drug to women, initially in preparations made from extracts of human placentas. In the 1940s, however, scientists worked out how to collect it from the urine of pregnant horses, and in 1942 a drug called Premarin, which takes its name from 'PREgnant MARes' urINe' (PMU), was approved by the FDA for the treatment of hot flushes. As the drug gained widespread popularity in the 1960s, more and more 'PMU farms' were needed to fulfil demand. Described as unspeakably cruel by many animal welfare charities, such farms see large breeds such as Belgian–quarter horse crosses impregnated and kept standing tethered in stalls for most of their eleven-month pregnancies, with rubber urine collection bags attached to them at all times, and their drinking water limited to ensure their urine is as high as possible in oestrogen. Once their foals are born, the mares nurse them for around four months and are then impregnated again, and they are kept on this cycle for around twelve years. Many of the foals and older mares are sold to the slaughterhouse. It's hard to establish the numbers of horses involved, in particular since production has moved to China following growing pressure around welfare, but a 2015 article cites 90,000 mares on so-called PMU farms,[3] and in 2020 in the US alone, there were more than 1 million prescriptions for Premarin.[4] If you want to be sure your brand of HRT does not have any part in this industry, ask your doctor (or Google) to make sure it does not contain so-called conjugated equine estrogens (CEE).

Aside from the issue of animal welfare, HRT has also been the subject of controversy because of concerns over the health risks to women. In the 1970s, links were established with endometrial cancer – because oestrogen on its own can stimulate the lining of the womb – and the dose was adjusted, and combined with progesterone. This is why, if you have not had a hysterectomy, you will still be prescribed 'combined HRT' today, a mix of oestrogen and progesterone; but if you no longer have a uterus, you can take oestrogen-only HRT. Then, in 1998, a large randomised study called the Women's Health Initiative (WHI) began and in 2002 published the first set of results, which showed an increased risk of coronary heart disease and breast cancer. In 2004, a second part of the WHI trial was stopped due to concerns over an increased risk of stroke, and alarm began to spread about HRT, with many women halting their use, and both doctors and women alike were left confused by the findings.[5] The results of the WHI trial continue to be debated to date, with some suggesting the study itself was flawed, some (including the WHI) claiming the concerns were over-estimated,[6] and others seeming to say 'that was then, this is now' and that the new 'bioidentical' HRT is safer, or even claiming that it has 'protective' health benefits beyond the alleviation of menopause symptoms, such as the prevention of osteoporosis,[7] a reduction in the risk of heart disease,[8] dementia,[9] and even potentially making you look 'younger' by improving your metabolism,[10] fat distribution, and maintaining collagen and skin elasticity.[11]

This chapter is not going to be a forensic analysis of the evidence around HRT, but suffice it to say, if you want to take it, you will be able to seek out evidence to support that decision, and if you'd rather not take it, you'll find evidence to say that's also a fair choice. Much of the evidence you will find is a mix of both, and depends on your age, your stage of menopause, the severity of your symptoms, the type of HRT you choose, and a variety of other factors.[12] In spite of bold claims, none of the evidence around HRT is conclusive; much more research is needed, in particular into the newer brands of bioidentical HRT – we just don't have the long-term studies on them yet. As with all choices, there are benefits and risks to every decision, and those benefits and risks will be unique to you – an individual with your own health history and lifestyle choices. Ultimately, whether or not you personally choose to take HRT and whether or not it works for you is not really the point. What is more interesting to me is the attitudes to the female body and to being female that surround the menopause rite of passage, and the sense of familiarity I feel when I see menopause presented as something awful that happens to women, with a whole list of dreadful symptoms, and a corresponding range of medical treatments to help them experience as little of it as possible. In spite of the limited understanding medical science has of the purpose and workings of the female body, we are nevertheless confidently presented with a branded drug or treatment for every stage. Menstruation, pregnancy and birth, and then menopause; each phase of our lives is explained to us as a problem to be fixed, a burden on both ourselves and others, and a set of 'symptoms'. Every function of a woman's body is, in fact, a malfunction – simply part of the unfortunate short straw we have drawn of being female, but panic not, each malfunction has a corresponding set of medical 'treatments' to alleviate 'symptoms'. As well as HRT, there are a variety of other treatments for menopause, including different drugs to reduce hot flushes; creams, tablets or rings containing oestrogen for vaginal dryness; anti-depressants (which are said to help with hot flushes as well as low mood); testosterone gel to boost sex drive; the Mirena coil, which releases progesterone into the uterus. Recent developments include ovarian tissue cryopreservation and transplantation (OTCT), a procedure costing up to £11,000, in which a slice of the ovary of a healthy young women is removed, cryopreserved and then regrafted into the pelvis or under the skin in the forearm later in life, with the aim of delaying their menopause.[13] In this way, menopause could be said to be highly 'medicalised', just like every other female biological experience. And just like every other female biological experience, it's also monetised, with the HRT industry alone predicted to be worth 50 billion US dollars globally by 2030, and many other companies and individuals, from pharma to holistic treatments, making big profits out of the menopause.[14]

But these are not the only parallels: just like menstruation, pregnancy and birth, menopause can also be reframed in similar ways. Some even describe it as 'second puberty', and while in some cases this definition only serves to further support the idea of it being something we'd all be better off without, others see it as a similar transformative rite of passage, difficult at times but necessary to experience in order to move into a new phase of our lives. There are parallels with childbirth, too, as we struggle, suffer, surrender, but ultimately produce a new human, not a baby this time, but a reinvention of ourselves. Teacher and expert in women's wisdom Jane Hardwicke Collings explores the direct links between each rite of passage: menarche, childbirth and menopause. With each of these life phases she feels we are offered an opportunity to learn about ourselves, and often to heal trauma and shame in our 'red thread' – the maternal line of our family (see page 63). If we can heal our relationship to menstruation, we may find that our approach to childbirth is different. Likewise through childbirth we are again offered an opportunity to transform our relationship to our bodies, and these transformations will show up for us again when our perimenopause time arrives. Each of these rites of passage can have a powerful impact, she explains, because 'what happens at these times informs us on a deep subliminal level of how our culture values the new role we are being initiated into and therefore how we are expected to behave in that role',[15] Jane even has a word for this time in women's lives, 'maga', which she describes as the phase 'after mother and before crone'.[16] 'Back in 2005 I was visiting a friend, Cedar Barstow, in Boulder, Colorado, and we were talking about the phases of the Triple

Goddess – maiden, mother and crone,' she tells me. 'Cedar explained that she felt, although her days in the full role of "mother" were over, she didn't feel she was ready for "crone" just yet! She was out in the world, doing her best work. She told me, 'I'm not wondering what I'm doing with my life any more. I'm doing it! I've arrived at my self!' Along with another woman in Cedar's community, Sylvia Keepers, she came to the name maga: the female version of magus, the wizard, wise man or magician. 'Women live a lot longer now than they did at the time the idea of three phases – maiden, mother, crone – was first relevant,' says Jane. 'It makes sense that they need this extra phase, before they are truly in old age, in a time when they are really at the peak of their powers and their confidence, truly in their stride. This is maga, the wise woman, the enchantress, the autumn woman and the harvest queen, enjoying the fruits of her life's labours.'

Feminine Forever

My initial feelings on being told that I might be 'peri' have since revealed to me a lot of the internalised disrespect I've been carrying all my life for older women. To put it in one simple sentence, my basic reaction was, '*I don't want to be that.*' But why? If Jane Hardwicke Collings is right that what happens at each female rite of passage informs us of how our culture now expects us to behave, then – speaking personally – I'd say that menarche taught me a certain level of shame and disgust in my female body; birth tried very hard (but eventually failed) to encourage self-sacrifice as I came to motherhood, and now

– menopause? Menopause seems to be telling me that being female and past fifty is 'as good as dead' in our culture, and that my only hope if I want to stay relevant is to medically maintain my oestrogen levels to match those of my younger self, and make use of as many fillers and filters as I can while I'm at it. As the old song goes, 'keep young and beautiful if you want to be loved'.[17] It's hardly surprising that I, like many other women, fear menopause and want, if possible, to be 'cured' of it, given the huge value placed on youth and beauty. We may not personally define ourselves on either our attractiveness or our fertility, but losing both lays bare for us just how many doors – literal and metaphorical – were opened for us on account of both. Just as in motherhood we may have felt our work of childcare devalued or unnoticed, or – as I did – that we were literally 'hidden' during long days and nights at home with our babies, now in menopause we may feel invisible again, but this time even as we walk down the street. In spite of having disliked the male gaze for decades, we may now feel a bit miffed that we are no longer noticed; as Germaine Greer puts it in *The Change*, 'Men lose interest in manipulating her femaleness: they no longer sniff around her . . . The change hurts. Like a person newly released from leg-irons, the freed woman staggers at first . . . For the first time in her life she finds that she has to raise her voice or wait endlessly while other people push in front of her.'[18] Celebrities in their fifties and beyond have recently begun to frame this time of life as empowering and liberating, for example Pamela Anderson who went make-up free at Paris Fashion Week in 2023 stating, 'I'm not trying to be the prettiest girl in the room. Why am I going to sit in the make-up chair for two hours when I could be at the Louvre? I could go look at some architecture. I could walk around Paris. There's so much to do at the flea market. I could do so many things.'

In our male-centred world, menopause is often framed as a problem not so much to women, but to the men who have to both live with us and look at us, and on occasion feel the sting of our rejection. Freud described it in 1913 as a time when a woman's character 'undergoes a peculiar alteration', and she becomes 'quarrelsome, vexatious, overbearing, petty and stingy'. Whether the loss of female libido that traditionally accompanies midlife is part of this complaint is perhaps a subject for an entirely separate book – suffice it to say, it's complicated. Original adverts for HRT certainly proclaimed that it was 'for husbands, too' and could make women 'pleasant to live with once again'.[19] Just over a hundred years later, Caitlin Moran explained this phenomenon from a female perspective in her column in *The Times* as a 'hormonal hangover', where women are effectively 'sobering up' after a few decades of being bathed in the softening effect of oestrogen.[20] Rather than making us angry, she says, menopause simply stops us being so forgiving. 'It's uncovered her actual personality and thoughts, under all the hormones . . . You don't want to be encouraging, loving and kind. Who, when sober, does?' Writing in the *New Statesman*, Suzanne Moore also describes this lack of enthusiasm for the middle ground that menopause brings: 'I don't really have the mood swings that some talk about. I have just the one mood. Rage. I am enraged as soon as I wake up, enraged by the news, enraged by how the world is, enraged when I can't sleep, and I can never sleep.'[21]

In a similar way to the 'pre-menstrual truth' of PMT, menopause removes both a layer of tolerance and our energy for self-censorship. We may find again the rolled eyes and accusations of being 'hormonal', often when we are simply stating our boundaries and our dissatisfaction with the status quo calmly and clearly. Doing so is not so much a problem for us, as for those we live with, who may be surprised to hear our sudden list of grievances, which are new to them but which we have been carefully storing up for some time. We may feel extremely angry – not a very acceptable emotion in females – and although this anger may shock those around us, it's quite possible that it's justified, given the burden of carework women carry, the mental load of family life, the pay gap, the sexual harassment, the lack of justice for perpetrators of violence and abuse of women . . . the list goes on. After fifty years of all this and more and with no sign of improvement, we may no longer feel like asking nicely for things to change. But this firm no, this decision to be actively less tolerant and much more assertive of our needs – expressed by many women as having 'zero fucks left to give' – is not very 'feminine' – and this appears to be another issue with menopausal women that men have highlighted, most notably the American doctor Robert Wilson in his 1966 book, *Feminine Forever*. The book, which would be quite hilarious if it weren't for the fact that 1966 really isn't that long ago in terms of attitude change, is quite clear: menopause is a 'crippling disease', and menopausal women are 'castrates', and 'no longer a woman, but a neuter'.[22]

Wilson is quite clear that there is one thing, and one thing only, that menopausal women need in order to restore their femininity – medical intervention in the form of hormone treatment. 'Women, after all, have the right to remain women,' he writes.

What Is a (Menopausal) Woman?

As it happens, it later emerged that *Feminine Forever,* and Wilson's own research foundation, were both backed by a major pharmaceutical company with a brand-new product to sell: HRT.[23] The book was a bestseller, and within a decade of its publication, the menopause drug of the day, Premarin (yes, the horse-urine one!), became the fifth most prescribed drug in the United States.[24] Wilson's message to a generation of women – and their doctors – was that HRT was an absolute necessity if they wished to 'remain feminine for life'. His suggestion, that without oestrogen we literally cease being women at all, is interesting – what a shame he didn't live to see that question being asked all the way to the Supreme Court: 'What *is* a woman?' Having read his book, I suspect his answer might boil down to the basics: appealing looks and submissive behaviour. But while his ideas may be hilariously outdated, nearly six decades later how far have we moved on? We find ourselves in a world in which 'gender' is increasingly performative, with heavily applied 'contouring' make-up, fake eyelashes, pink handbags and heels, and even a hairless 'Barbie' vulva, all signifying 'woman'. Historic female figures who defied the restrictions placed on women or who dressed as men to escape them – such as Guanyin,[25] Joan of Arc,[26] and

Queen Hatshepsut of Egypt – have been declared transgender, while modern butch lesbians face suggestions that, because they dress in a way that is gender non-conforming, they must actually be men.[27] We have influencers like Dylan Mulvaney, a person born male but who has publicly documented their gender transition on social media, and now likes dresses and dolls and skipping through flower meadows in heels, all of which are apparently part of 'girlhood'. Dylan tells us of dreams to be a 'trophy wife': '. . . they can picture me walking down the aisle to be their trophy bride . . . I would totally be good at that, don't you think? "*Dinner's ready! Yoo-hoo!*"' Mulvaney certainly ticks a lot of boxes for Robert Wilson's definition of 'feminine' and, ideologically at least, would arguably be great wife material for another high-profile influencer, Andrew Tate, known for his brand of misogynistic hypermasculinity in which 'the women belong to the man', and are 'the ultimate status symbol', as long as they are young and pretty and agree with everything he says. For all that we may laugh at *Feminine Forever*, here in 2026 we seem to be drifting back towards its binary values – and where does that leave the menopausal woman? Flat shoes, loose-fitting clothes, soft, sagging skin and the odd stray hair on her chin, no longer fertile, frequently angry and unapologetically assertive – is she still 'feminine'? Is she still a woman? Whatever she is, she seems to upset the forces of patriarchy and will frequently be seen being undermined with agist tropes – 'Karen', 'dinosaur', 'harridan' – and even (and I've witnessed this often on social media) being accused of looking either like a man or a trans woman. This is of course meant in the same age-old derogatory way that Robert Wilson would no doubt have approved of.

Perhaps it is no coincidence that in these times of women being increasingly defined by their adherence (or lack of it) to hyperfemininity, we are more in love with HRT than ever. Women are still being peddled the old idea that menopause is nothing more than a list of negative symptoms that HRT can potentially fix, coupled with a new, 'empowering', twenty-first-century idea that, with the help of HRT, we can continue to 'kick ass'. In England, the number of prescriptions for HRT has risen by 35 per cent since 2022.[28] Davina McCall and Dr Naomi Potter's bestselling *Menopausing* is one of several influential books and podcasts credited with influencing this uptick,[29] which has even been branded the 'Davina effect'.[30] The book contains multiple first-hand accounts from women of how they became a 'shadow of themselves' before taking oestrogen, including Davina herself, who says, 'HRT helped me rediscover myself. I had disappeared, and now I'm back.' HRT, she says, is a 'GIANT leap for womankind. And, in fact, mankind. And, in fact, allkind – because when we're OK, everyone's OK . . . HRT is completely transformative. It does not just delay your menopause, it puts you back where you were.' A bit like the original HRT marketing of *Feminine Forever*, the message is that there is something *restorative* about oestrogen, and in order for this messaging to work, there has to be, lurking somewhere underneath, in the shadows, the idea that menopause is essentially something wrong with women – a loss, a negative change or even a catastrophe – that needs to be put right.

The idea that HRT can 'put us back where we were' is very tempting to anyone in their mid-forties. Who doesn't want to stop or even rewind the clock, in particular as it begins to tick ever louder? We live in a world that prizes youth over age, and in which an older woman on the catwalk, in a leading role or on the cover of a magazine (in particular one who isn't fillered or filtered, who actually 'looks her age') is still rare enough to make headlines. But we cannot go back to where we were. We cannot be 'feminine' forever, if feminine means fertile and glowy and energised and shaggable. In fact, we cannot be anything 'forever', because we cannot 'be' forever. We are mortal. We are ageing. Our lives of seven or eight decades or so, are not particularly long, and – for every single human without exception – they will end. Not only that, but as my then 12-year-old daughter put it to me when she was having her own dark realisations, there will come a time when there is nobody alive who remembers us. Yes, I thought, but I didn't tell her that there is even a word for this: 'memory death'. Each of us has two deaths – our actual death, and then our memory death, which happens when the last person alive who remembers us dies. As children come to their teenage years they begin to contemplate all of this, and take to their rooms, listening to music in headphones and looking miserable and troubled. 'Hormones,' we say. In mid-life, the bell tolls again. The reality that time is slipping away hits us each time we look in the mirror. We have made some choices by now. Were they the right ones? What if? How many years might we have left? How old will we be when our children are the age we are now? Is it too late to . . .? And so on. We wake in the night with these thoughts, and can't get back to sleep. We are told: 'Hormones.'

The Body-Mind in Menopause

My reaction to being told I was perimenopausal – '*I don't want to be that*' – seems perfectly reasonable when you consider that '*that*' is not only an ageing woman who is no longer considered relevant or even visible by her immediate culture, but also a person for whom time is running out, a person who is 'over the hill' and sliding rapidly down the other side towards the one rite of passage we don't get to write about afterwards: death. As our perimenopausal hormones rage, rather like our teenage daughters we can be quick to anger. But anger can very often be a sign of something else, deeper under the surface: unexpressed grief. In both puberty and menopause, we are losing something: in puberty, childhood; in menopause, youth and fertility. Telling both teens and perimenopausal women that our feelings are simply an unfortunate side effect of our sex, a sort of unpleasant emotional waste product, diminishes the complexity of our life transition. It also exacerbates it by continuing to encourage us to keep a lid on our feelings, adding to the pressure cooker of our rage. In our forties and fifties, there can be much to grieve, beyond our youth and fertility. We may lose parents or watch them become ill or frail, often, as women, carrying the responsibility for their care. If we have children we may notice them begin to need us much less at this time, we may have problems in our relationships with them or they may 'fly the nest'. We may divorce (mid-forties is the most common age for marriage break-up), and – just as we are often coming to feel at the peak of our abilities and expertise – we may feel sidelined in the workplace as the gender pay gap reaches its widest point, with women in their forties and fifties earning 20 per cent less than their male peers.[31] All of this grief needs a place to go, and in a world that still prefers us to keep our sorrow hidden away, it can instead manifest as snappiness, frustration, resentment, hostility, anger and searing, white-hot rage. Ask a fuming-mad perimenopausal woman (or, if that woman is you, ask yourself), 'What are you sad about?' and see what happens.

The more difficult psychological aspects of menopause are only just beginning to be discussed. We know that the highest rates of suicide among women are in the 45- to 54-year-old age group, and that these have risen 6 per cent in the last twenty years.[32] The risk of serious depression is significantly increased in perimenopause,[33] and a 2022 survey of 2,000 women commissioned by the House of Commons Women and Equalities Select Committee found 69 per cent reported feeling some level of anxiety or depression.[34] Hormones certainly play a role: women who have experienced poor mental health in relation to other periods of fluctuating hormones (for example, those who've suffered premenstrual mood disorders or postpartum depression) are more at risk of serious depression in menopause.[35] As does diet – our modern ultra processed fare has been shown to have a powerful negative impact on women's mid-life mental health. However, what seems to happen in perimenopause is a perfect storm of fluctuating hormones alongside psychosocial factors, such as lack of support and existential crisis, and health factors, such as tiredness, poor diet and alcohol misuse. In a similar way to the change we experience when we have our first baby, menopause is a complex and tough psychological and physical transition.

To each transition of the matriflux we bring our own personal history, and this will impact us in ways that only a person anxious to avoid the painful complexity of their own or another's emotional life would attempt to explain as simply 'hormonal'. The body and mind are connected parts of a whole; a physical experience can be immensely psychologically damaging and painful just as it can be life-enhancing, and the physical experiences of menarche, childbirth and menopause may bring us into contact with our sexed bodies in ways that are triggering and deeply uncomfortable. Researchers have found that a history of early childhood maltreatment is highly prevalent among those women seeking help for difficult menopausal symptoms, and that these women are also more likely to suffer depression around menopause.[36] One study found that girls who experienced adverse childhood experiences (these can be all types of abuse and neglect) could be up to twice as likely to suffer depression in perimenopause, while another study found that women with a physical or sexual abuse history had approximately 1.5 to 2 times the number of sleep vasomotor symptoms (hot flushes and night sweats) of women without this history.[37] Researchers have also found that girls who are sexually abused in childhood will begin puberty and have their first period earlier – as much as a year before their non-abused peers, and also that childhood experiences of physical abuse can lead to a delayed menarche.[38]

In the same way, women who have been exposed to sexual abuse or violence, or who have witnessed violence and abuse against their own children, will reach menopause over eight years earlier, according to a 2022 study.[39] It is thought that it is the impact of extreme stress that instigates both early menarche and menopause in these groups of women, both of which put them at risk of other mental and physical health problems. Given the extent of the physical and sexual abuse of women and girls – as many as one in five girls are sexually abused,[40] and the WHO estimates that one in three women globally will be subjected to physical or sexual violence in their lifetime – it is somewhat extraordinary that we largely continue to ignore the ways in which this may impact on female biological experiences.[41]

A holistic approach to women's health would require us to join up the dots between body and mind, throughout the female lifespan, something that our highly medicalised culture is simply not in the habit of doing. Women who try hypnobirthing in pregnancy are still thought of as somewhat on the lunatic fringe, which is why, in *The Positive Birth Book*, I used a lot of analogies with elite sportspeople when I wrote a section about the body–mind connection. Somehow, when an (often male) athlete says they use a technique called 'positive self-talk' we find it more acceptable than when a pregnant woman talks about 'affirmations', but the two are one and the same. Our mindset and our expectations can shape our reality: everyone knows that Muhammad Ali said, 'I am the greatest,' but not everyone remembers his next line: 'I said that even before I knew I was.' When it comes to menopause, marketing it as a disease is an incredibly lucrative business – the global HRT market was valued at 24.88 billion dollars in 2021 and is expected to reach nearly 50 billion dollars by 2030.[42] To maintain this market, however, consistent focus must be given to unpleasant symptoms, ageing and loss of femininity, shaping our expectations almost entirely negatively. It is positively lucrative for HRT manufacturers to encourage and maintain the negative narrative. But researchers have found that how we feel about this life transition has a profound influence: women who have negative expectations of menopause will report more symptoms,[43] and women tend to have worse experiences of menopause in countries where their value is linked to youth and reproductive capacity and ageing is associated with decline.[44] Conversely, cultures in which menopause signifies a transition to a higher status tend not to attribute a list of difficult symptoms to it. First Nations women in Canada, for example, were said by researchers not to 'conceptually link' menopause to 'symptoms typical of menopause from a medical perspective' and did not even have a word for 'menopause'.[45] Instead, they explained that they simply saw it as the end of menstruation, and had been told about it from childhood. Although they experienced some symptoms, such as hot flushes and mood swings, overall they felt they were beginning to be perceived as 'respected . . . a woman with wisdom', 'not elderly as in old and grey and wrinkled, but old and wise'. 'In our belief, we hold the woman very sacred; she is the life giver,' they explained, and they welcomed this new status. Similarly, Mayan women report very few negative effects of menopause, but instead see it as the time of the acquisition of a new status of community leader, spiritual elder, healer and wise woman.[46] In Māori culture, they speak of *ruahine*, which translates as 'second woman', meaning the second season of a woman's life, but also means 'woman of importance' or 'wise woman', signifying a time of increased respect and responsibility in the community.[47] Māori woman Michelle Uriarau told me, 'It is usually only *kuia* [post-menopausal female elders] that can perform *karanga* [ceremonial welcome] onto the *marae*. Additionally *only wāhine* [women] can *karanga* – not men – and because of this, the woman's voice is the first voice to be heard.' In Traditional Chinese medicine, menopause is referred to as the 'second spring', a time when, because we have ceased menstruating, our blood and our *qi* (energy) is instead directed to our heart, where our *shén*, or spirit, resides. This shift in our *qi* allows us to access new levels of courage, vibrancy and creativity.[48]

Widening our view to look cross-culturally reinforces that there is no universal menopause experience. Hot flushes and night sweats are far more prevalent among women in the US and Europe than in Asia[49]; one study found that only 5 per cent of women in Indonesia reported hot flushes, with the women there instead being far more likely to report joint aches and pains as their main symptom.[50] Until recently, there was no word for 'hot flush' in Japanese. Menopause there is referred to as *konenki*, which translates as 'time/season/energy of renewal and regeneration' – a contrast to our own word menopause, which simply translates as 'monthly – cease', or the end of our periods. Since words say so much about mindset and therefore experience, perhaps we ought to return to the more old-fashioned word for menopause, climacteric, meaning a critical life period of remarkable change, with its roots in the Greek *klimakter*, meaning 'rung of a ladder'.

Women in Japan have the longest life expectancy in the world, low rates of heart disease and cancer, and a diet that is very different from the highly processed food of their Western counterparts; low in meat, dairy products and sugar, and high in fish, vegetables and soybeans. Some research suggests that this soy consumption may affect oestrogen levels and hormone balance (soy is one of the plants they use to make bioidentical HRT); however, the reason for an easier menopause in Japan is unlikely to be just one thing.[51] The medical anthropologist Margaret Lock uses the term 'local biologies' to convey how the human bodily experience of something as universal as menopause can vary so much depending on geography, with its infinite combination of expectations, culture, history, diet, lifestyle and mindset.[52] Looking globally, we can see menopause through a wider lens, and then turn this lens back on ourselves and our own lives. Just as we should if we experience problems when we are menstruating or pregnant, if menopause symptoms are problematic we should consider all options: are we eating plenty of fresh and unprocessed foods? How is our mindset? What about our mental health? Do we have unresolved trauma or grief? How are we sleeping? Are we happy? What about exercise – are we doing too much, or too little? Do we smoke or take drugs? What about alcohol – have we tried life without it for a while? Do we drink enough water? Do we feel loved? Do we take any time for ourselves? Do we get enough hugs? In short, instead of focusing on what menopause is bringing to us, we need to turn the lens on what we are bringing to menopause. All of this can be explored alongside HRT, or without it. We need a much more holistic approach.

Menopause as a Return

There is soul work to be done at this time in our lives, whether we choose HRT or not. A facing-up to our mortality and impermanence, an exploration of what youth and our culture's definition of beauty have meant to us, a mourning of our losses, a reassessement of both our relationship with our female bodies and our femininity, and a refocusing of our sense of purpose, as well as broadening our thinking about menopause as a rite of passage into a newer, stronger and more powerful version of ourselves. This idea of menopause as an upgrade rather than 'the beginning of the end' is a fruitful reframe; a new start; the beginning of our 'Queenage'; and the birth of a new version of ourselves: the wise woman.

On the other hand, all of these imply a linear version of life, a constant movement forwards. Sometimes this concept can become tiring, as hidden within it is the implication that we must always be working on ourselves as a project, and that if we are not feeling and celebrating our personal 'growth' on the daily, we may need a course, a supplement, a retreat, a book, a guru.

But the matriflux is not linear – it's a cycle. As such, perhaps we could consider a third way of thinking about menopause – not as an ending, *or* as an upgrade, but as a return. A cyclical 'looping back' in which we rediscover the core person we were, before fertility happened.

As women, fertility – whether or not we have children – is an exciting gift. I currently see it blooming in my teenage daughters and I notice how it opens up their world and energises them to seek adventure, company, excitement and, yes, sex. But the flip side of this – and what they and none of us realise at the time, of course – is that the whole thing is going to knock them off course and into entirely new orbits, for the next couple of decades at least. And that much of this will probably involve a setting aside of their own needs, hopes, desires.

Oestrogen, in some ways, derails us. It softens our judgement and encourages a more forgiving nature. It blinds us to faults. It urges us to reproduce. Under oestrogen's spell, we obey, only to feel shocked at the scene that surrounds us when menopause shakes us roughly awake. For many of us, some of the struggle of 'The Change' is focused on regret: *why did I do that? what was I thinking?* We look at the choices we've made and where they've led us with fresh eyes, and many of us feel awakened to a sense we've been exploited, and determined to be a lot less tolerant. No wonder Robert Wilson, as well as countless other doctors and mental health experts, have explored a variety of ways to numb women of this age and put them firmly back to sleep.

Amidst this time of revision, I also feel a sense of return. Who was that girl in the 1980s, what were her priorities, what were her dreams, before puberty changed her? I remember being her. I remember walking up the little side lane near my house and spending a long time just looking into the hedge and watching baby birds in a nest. I remember my deep, never-ending, sibling-like love for my labrador Ben. I remember playing at libraries and arranging books in neat rows. I remember waking early every morning and tearing through detective stories, spy stories, magical stories, any stories I could get my hands on. I read as if there were no time left.

At that point I had no limits on my sense of what I could become. Nor did I particularly think about what I *would* become, because for the most part, I was absorbed in the present moment, and carefree. When adults asked what I wished to be when I grew up, my answer would depend on what book character I'd most recently fallen in love with: I'd be a nurse, a show jumper, a stable boy, a detective, I really had no idea. Mostly I just wanted to be just a couple of years older than I actually was and heading in a horse and carriage towards a big house where my adventure would begin.

Pre-puberty Milli was called Melinda. Some of the work of menopause, I feel, is to reconnect with that girl. In my twenties, life was intensely occupied by the complex quest to find 'the one'. In my thirties, it was occupied by small children and my every waking and sleeping moment was crowded and interrupted. Suddenly now my children don't need me as fiercely and intensely; I have space. Any mum reading this will know what that simple sentence means: *I have space.* Yes yes, I know, now I'm supposed to say how much I miss those little, needy people. Well, I don't actually. I miss the idea of them. The reality was bloody hard work and I feel more like: yes, it was lovely, but been there, done that, got the T-shirt.

There is a 'what now' feeling about this time of life. There is a pressure to 'grow', but what if we already 'are'. Rather than becoming someone new, maybe we simply need to return to the person we always were, before love, sex, motherhood and oestrogen distracted us? Who was that core person; what pleased her; what were her needs? Were there dreams she had that are yet to be fulfilled? Were there activities she enjoyed that have long been abandoned? Now, there is space for her again. But who was she then, and who is she now?

Returning, we do not always find things as we left them. I remember once coming back from a holiday to discover a starling had been trapped for several days in my kitchen. It had survived by pecking away at the contents of the fruit bowl, shitting liberally everywhere, and flapping around the worktops sending glassware flying to smash in large quantities across the floor. Adult Milli found this to be a bit of a nightmare; Melinda would have found it a great adventure and decided immediately to adopt the starling as a pet and teach it to talk.

Coming back to my core self now I am not and will never be that 10-year-old, daydreaming wistfully and wondering how hard she would have to practice to learn as many animal languages as Dr Doolittle. Life has wreaked its havoc. But under the broken glass and the rotted fruit peel and the shit, something of her remains. As a mum, I have seen first-hand how children hatch out of the egg with a ready-formed personality and a plan. My task now is to remember mine.

Chapter 7

Crone Myths

'Change
Said the sun to the moon,
You cannot stay.
Change
Says the moon to the waters,
All is flowing.'

KATHLEEN RAINE, *Change*

Every rite of passage has a so-called liminal stage or threshold, where things get pretty intense. It's like everything is being broken down, and although this has to happen in order for there to be renewal and change, at the time it can feel chaotic or filled with drama and uncertainty. There's a bunch of predictable metaphors we could bring in here. The mythical phoenix, a beautiful firebird, only one of which can exist in the world at a time, builds her nest of aromatic twigs and spices, sets it alight and is consumed by the flames, only to regenerate or be born anew from the fire. The caterpillar, who surely does not know what fate awaits her, dissolves and digests to soup inside the cocoon, apart from the 'imaginal discs' – groups of cells that contain all the instructions needed to make the butterfly. In ritual, humans recreate these transitional states:

first, by preparing themselves or the space, perhaps by putting on special clothes or burning incense or clearing the area to be used, then, by entering into the ritual itself, during which they usually behave in a different way to normal, and finally, by emerging and returning to their usual lives, transformed. A wedding is, of course, a perfect example of this, but there are many others, from ceremonies with dancing or drugs to induce trance-like states, to fire festivals such as Guy Fawkes Night, to the roaring of familiar songs at a sports game, to the reciting of blessings and the lighting of candles in most major world religions. The patterns of these rituals that humans around the world construct in order to make meaning replicate the various transitions of the matriflux, each of which has its time of preparation, its liminal phase as the threshold is crossed, and its return following transformation. When my 12-year-old daughter was at the threshold of puberty, I watched her circling, resisting, preparing and gathering herself as she prepared to make the crossing. One day she would brush the hair of all of her dolls and line them up carefully; the next day try out eyeshadows. Then, as she reached menarche, there was a period of both celebration and adjustment. I remember, too, the liminal stage in each of my three labours, a part of which is literally called 'transition', where you have reached a deeply altered, trance-like state and you are not sure if you can go on. It feels as if the universe is cracking apart and your own body is splitting in half, too, as you pause, teetering on the brink, filled with uncertainty – and then roar your baby into the world, and a new version of yourself along with them. Perimenopause is another liminal phase, at the end of which we cross another threshold, one year after our final period, into menopause. Technically speaking, menopause is only one day – after which, we are, for the rest of our lives, a 'post-menopausal' woman. Unless we take HRT and take it forever (as some women will), then our oestrogen and progesterone levels will settle, we will no longer have hormonal ups and downs, and any 'symptoms' associated with these should also cease. Hormonally, at least, we return to a similar experience of our pre-pubescent selves: we no longer 'cycle'.

In many myths and stories, the protagonist 'descends', sometimes into a dark place, which at the time feels challenging and hopeless. The ancient Sumerian poem *The Descent of Inanna,* composed around 2100–1900 BCE, is thought to be the oldest surviving complete narrative with a goddess as the central character. Inanna, who like Mary is known as 'Queen of Heaven', dresses in her fine clothes and gold and heads down to visit her sister Ereshkigal, Queen of Darkness, in the shadowy underworld known as the Kur. To get in, Inanna must pass through seven gates, and at each one, another layer of her finery is removed and taken from her, until she finally stands before her sister, naked. Filled with rage, Ereshkigal turns her sister Inanna into a rotting piece of meat, and she is hung by a hook on the wall. Before Inanna made her descent, however, she had instructed her servant Ninshubur to come to her aid if she did not return. Ninshubur appeals to the sky gods, and finally one of them, Enki, sends help in the form of two little figures made from the dirt beneath his fingernails. This pair revive the corpse of Inanna with food and water, and she makes her ascent. A deal must still be struck, however, and Ereshkigal insists that someone should be chosen to take Inanna's place. On her return, Inanna finds her husband, Dumuzid, who, instead of mourning her loss as others are, is dressed in his finery and relaxing on *her* throne! Well, what would you do? That's right – she chooses Dumuzid, and off he is dragged to the Kur, although, eventually, Dumuzid's sister persuades Inanna to be compassionate and a compromise is reached – Dumuzid must spend only half the year in the underworld and the other half with Inanna. Thus the myth explains the seasons, in a similar way to another story of descent and rising, the Greek myth of Persephone, although there is clearly much, much more to the story than this.

Inanna rises again, but she is changed. As the first line of the ancient poem tells us, 'From the Great Above, she opened her ear to the Great Below.' Inanna listens in to the shadow. By making herself vulnerable, by shedding some of the trappings of her life, descending and facing death itself, she becomes more multi-dimensional on her return. Her story resonates with many female life experiences, but perhaps none more so than the descent of perimenopause, the listening in and confronting of the darkness at this time, and the rising, transformed and empowered, which can happen when our cycles have ended.

Sharon Blackie, in her book *Hagitude: Reimagining the Second Half of Life*, compares menopause to the phase of alchemy known as *Nigredo*, a 'blackening' during which it was believed the substance being transformed suffered greatly as it was forced to shed unnecessary layers and reveal its true nature. Alchemists call this 'mortification', which means 'facing the dead parts', and the first stage of this is 'calcination', which means, 'reduced to the bone by burning'. Blackie compares this to the fire of menopause, the anger, the hot flushes, and asks, 'What is all that fire for, during menopause? As with the process of calcination, it's to burn away the dead parts of our lives so that we can reveal the buried treasure within.' It's a time when we need to ask hard questions about the entire structure of our lives, and if we don't feel they're going to support us or nourish us in the next phase, well, it's time to burn them down.

The Fire Reclaimed

Siobhan Daniels was working in a successful job at the BBC during her fifties but feeling overwhelmed with life. 'I was broken – with menopause, family bereavements, empty nest as my daughter had left home, and being marginalised and made to feel voiceless at work,' she told me. 'I just did not want to carry on living the way that I was living. I was disillusioned with the way everybody, including me, was working long hours, and earning lots of money to buy lots of stuff. I was working ten-hour days and filling my home with beautiful things and doing dinner parties, but it was stopping me from living and stopping me from being happy.' And then one morning, and she has no idea why, the idea of a motorhome popped into her head. As she headed towards her retirement at sixty, she made plans that astonished everyone who knew her – to sell everything she owned and hit the road. 'Now, after six years of living my nomadic life in my motorhome, I have found me and I like me. I have found my inner voice and my inner warrior. I am the mistress of my own destiny and I love that.' Siobhan runs an Instagram account and has written a book, *Retirement Rebel*, about her adventures and positive ageing, describing herself as 'ageless and fearless'. She's now planning to drive solo from Vancouver to Alaska. 'I think a lot of women repurpose their lives when in their mid-fifties – they want adventure. I am trying to show these women, there is so much more next! When you retire, you refire!'

Not all of Siobhan's 'refiring' has been easy or painless, though – in her book she writes about some 'dark nights of the soul'; for example, the time when she went out to the edge of a Scottish loch in the dark and screamed, letting go of a lot of her grief for lost family members. 'I was conscious that I hadn't dealt with what had pushed me to be doing this adventure in the first place,' she says. 'So I went out in the middle of the night to the edge of the water, and just screamed and shouted and had the conversations with my father – because I'd had a difficult childhood – with my colleagues at work who I wish I'd said certain things to; I grieved my brother and sister; I grieved my mother; I just dropped to my knees and was sobbing, and everything came out. Then all of a sudden I just got this overwhelming feeling of calmness, and I just thought, *That's it now, leave that behind and use it as fire in your belly to move forward, and inspire other people.* I don't have that anger about my past any more; in fact, I've even found ways to really love my father. I've come to terms with a lot of things through that night. So I would recommend screaming like a banshee at the edge of a loch to anybody.'

Other women describe this mix in their fifties and sixties of an exciting new lease of life, alongside mourning, anger and grief. Suzie Love, age 53, from Kent, found menopause a huge challenge, which has brought her to a new place. 'About three years ago I felt almost non-verbal with grief,' she told me. 'I felt my body was failing me and I was trying to support everyone around me, as so many women do. I also felt complete and utter despair and rage at the way women are treated. HRT helped a lot, as did giving up alcohol, as did respecting myself as I am and saying no a lot. I have now made so many positive changes. I make time for yoga every day, I take myself on solo adventures. I am a bolder, less apologetic woman and feel that age and the menopause has liberated me.' Vickie Curtis, also 53 and also feeling suddenly free, is making a new start at art college this autumn, after 'a lifetime behind a desk' as a management consultant, academic and, lastly, in the civil service. 'Getting to this stage of life prompted a lot of thinking – about what I wanted from life and what was important,' she explained. 'The pandemic exacerbated this, I think, and also prompted me to take a local art class. I've enrolled in a fine art foundation course and feel daunted, but now realise this is a good thing! I have found this experience and this stage of life incredibly liberating. I don't feel driven to please others, or to prove myself. I feel happy in my own skin for perhaps the first time in my life. At the same time I feel a lot of anger about how little has changed for women and girls. I'm hoping art might be a way for me to express this.' As a character called the Menopause Banshee puts it in the Netflix animation *Big Mouth*, 'This next chapter's yours to live, now you have no fucks to give.' As oestrogen, which some call the 'people-pleasing hormone', dips, we are no longer so willing to put ourselves last, and we have a new-found, healthy aggression. As women, we perhaps don't tend to think of aggression as healthy, but listening to the ways in which post-menopausal women seem to harness their anger and transform it into a determination to make positive changes seems to challenge this.

Female socialisation – in which girls and young women from an early age are taught to be passive, risk-averse and unchallenging, is well documented. As a parent for the last fifteen years I have observed it most vividly in the clothing departments of high-street stores, in which the T-shirts I can buy for my son are emblazoned with messages about space travel, computing and adventure, but those for my daughters carry slogans like 'Be Kind', 'Sunshine and Smiles' and 'Good Vibes Only'. The division of the sexes into girly pink and practical blue shocked me when my first daughter was small, and I dressed her in clothes from the boys section at times, simply because comfy trousers and dark-coloured tops were better suited to the tree climbing and puddle jumping that I thought every pre-schooler, regardless of their sex, should be doing. My efforts may perhaps have been in vain, though, so powerful is the culture my daughters are growing up in, and it might be that they, like so many other generations of women before them, will be post-menopausal before they are able to begin to break free of the gendered behaviours society expects of them. There are deep roots, too, to the fear that women can feel when they contemplate non-conformity; as Lucy H. Pearce writes in her book *Burning Woman*, 'Women, it seems, have an innate knowing of what it means to burn . . . and be burned. They know the dangers in their bones. And it makes them wary.' In the fifteenth and sixteenth centuries, conservative estimates suggest tens of thousands of women were tried for witchcraft and put to death across Europe, usually by being burned at the stake, and scholars believe that the majority were older women of at least forty.[1] Although we may think of witch-hunts as historic, the charity Age International reports that the killing of older women accused of witchcraft continues, all over the world, from Ghana to India, Bangladesh and beyond. One woman who had been accused of witchcraft in Tanzania told Age International, 'Many people have the attitude that when a woman ages she becomes a witch. The mentality is that "old" means "witch".'[2] In the UK, 'invisibility, devaluation and derision towards the older woman is added to everyday misogyny', according to Karen Ingala Smith, creator of the Femicide Census.[3] In 2020, the census found that, of the 120 women killed in the UK that year by men, 50 per cent of the victims were 46 or older.[4]

In everyone's collective imagination lives the witch, the hag, the scold, the nag, the fishwife, the crone, the old biddy. We all know what this archetype signifies: unloved, outcast, weird, ugly, aged, and often, too strong in her views and with too much to say. Her hair is grey, her face warty, her teeth yellow, her hands gnarled. She meets none of the criteria for what author Victoria Smith calls 'Triple F Womanhood': fertile, feminine and fuckable. She lives alone, at the edge of the village or further into the woods, perhaps with a cat or two, and is often skilled in the ways of 'wortcunning' – the knowledge of the healing power of plants. Children fear her. She is the stuff of fairy tales, like Baba Yaga from Slavic folklore, who lives deep in the forest in a magical house on chicken legs, flies around in a pestle and mortar, sometimes providing aid to visitors but equally eating those who displease her after cooking them in her oven. She is found in the myths of every culture and is always wise and powerful, like the Cailleach in Gaelic myth, known in Scotland as Beira, a divine hag and ancient queen of winter, who made the mountains and the landscape itself. Women over fifty or sixty can share some of the qualities of Baba Yaga or the Cailleach – beholden to no one; powerful in their independence; disinterested in being 'nice'. They are highly disruptive to the patriarchal definition of femininity, and quietly but firmly out of control, which perhaps explains their centuries-long history of persecution. Utterly unafraid to burn you in her oven, the modern day Baba Yaga may conduct her roastings metaphorically on X instead and be called a 'Karen', a 'dinosaur' or a 'TERF', all of which, as Victoria Smith points out, are simply new iterations of 'hag hate', and clear attempts by patriarchy to undermine and control us. Indeed, such women are all the more despised because, rather than being fictional or historic, they have the temerity to be real and to live among us: 'When I picture today's hag,' writes Smith, 'I don't see someone who is an easily defined outsider, neat to categorise and ripe for rehabilitation, but someone who inhabits an uneasy space between perfectly mundane and beyond the pale. She's not called Maleficent or Serafina or Elphaba, but Sharon or Carol or, yes, Karen . . .

We love the idea of the outspoken, boundary-defying woman in stories, rather than in the (ageing, decaying) flesh.' The hag, both ancient and modern, is feared because she represents both death and power, growth and destruction; she is seemingly unnecessary and at the same time invaluable. She is alarming and repulsive and yet, without her, there would be no life.

Pod Leaders

When it comes to post-menopausal women, anthropologists and biologists have a somewhat jarring unanswered question: why are these women still alive? Apparently they don't mean to be rude – they're simply thinking about it from an evolutionary perspective, the basics of which are: the purpose of survival is reproduction, and therefore, to outlive your fertility, potentially by several decades, is something of a puzzle. Basically, what is the point of a woman who can't make any more babies? As a post-menopausal woman myself, this question feels more than a little insulting. I'm pretty sure there *is* a point to my existence, and I think my three children would agree, if only because I'm the only one who knows the password to the screentime app. And even though I understand the evolutionary theory that underpins the question, it does come across a bit, 'You still here, luv?' particularly in light of centuries of cultural prejudice against older women that calls into question their existence when they no longer pass the Triple F challenge. It also strikes me as interesting that, when it comes to menopause, why women outlive it seems to be 'the big question'. Another question that might be equally interesting to ask is, what is the point of sex after menopause? After all, if infertile post-menopausal women are pointless from an evolutionary perspective, then surely having sex with them is equally pointless, too? But if you start googling that, it doesn't seem like any researchers have looked into it, and all you will find is a lot of articles telling women how many benefits there are to having sex at this age, and a raft of tips on how to get in the mood if they don't fancy it. Hmmm. It's almost as if the narrative is written by people who don't quite understand the point of women over 55 but want to keep having sex with them anyway.

The point of sex, of course, goes far beyond reproduction – we humans use it throughout our adult lives for a variety of reasons, from bonding to comfort to lust. Even before menopause, we are only fertile for a small window of a few days each month around ovulation, and yet we are sexually active throughout the menstrual cycle. Most women are familiar with idea of the 'biological clock', and the fact that our fertility begins to decline around our mid-thirties.[5] The idea that we are 'born with all of our eggs' and that we therefore gradually 'run out of eggs' is the most widely accepted, although this has been challenged in recent years, in particular by Jonathan Tilly, a reproductive biologist at Harvard, who has suggested that stem cells in the ovary may be capable of producing new eggs.[6] However, this remains largely theoretical, and has not yet been demonstrated to occur naturally in women. Whether we 'run out' or 'cease production', however, either way most of us will have many 'egg-free' years, which makes us unusual in that almost every other living creature is fertile until the very end, with the exception – as far as we currently understand – only of orcas (also known as killer whales), short-finned pilot whales, belugas and narwhals.[7] Various theories have been put forward to explain this human anomaly. Could it be that we simply live longer than we are intended to, perhaps because of our modern healthcare systems and rich and varied diets?[8] Or maybe, as evolutionary geneticists from Canada's McMaster University suggested in 2013, menopause has evolved because men are far more attracted to younger women – our genes literally mutating in response to men's lack of interest in us as we age, and our ovaries correspondingly shrivelling.[9] And yes, before you ask, the authors of that particular study were all male. Cheers, lads!

The most popular theory about why we women live so long without the ability to reproduce is the 'grandmother hypothesis'. Put simply, this suggests that menopause is an evolutionary adaptation, allowing us to give all our energy and focus from mid-life onwards to our existing children (it is sometimes also known as the 'mother hypothesis') and grandchildren, to make it more likely that our own genes will survive. Our own fertility as mothers drops off at around the same time that our daughters may be reaching reproduction age and may therefore need our support (although this has shifted in recent decades due to women having babies later in life), which may have evolved as a form of natural selection in times when food was scarce. Therefore, according to American anthropologist Kristen Hawkes, who was the first to gather evidence for the grandmother hypothesis, we are not actually 'post-reproductive', because we are still investing in the reproduction of our genes.[10] And this investment is effective: Hawkes's studies of the Hadza people of Tanzania found that the presence of a grandmother – in the Hadza's case as an extra pair of hands to forage food – boosted a child's chance of survival.[11] Another study into seventeenth- and eighteenth-century settlers in French Québec found that women whose mothers were still alive gave birth to more children, more of whom survived to adulthood, and that the closer these women lived to their mothers, the greater the chances of grandchild survival.[12] Grandmothers are also a repository for knowledge – in humans this may be the 'grandmother wisdom' of pregnancy, breastfeeding, childcare, herbs and healing, hunting and foraging, all of which are important for survival. In orca grandmothers, this knowledge seems to be primarily of salmon location hotspots, with post-menopausal orcas often found swimming at the front of their pod, leading their families to the best fishing locations.[13] Orca mothers also have a special relationship with their sons, who swim near them for most of their lives, and researchers at the University of Exeter have found that the longer an orca mother lives, the better her son's survival chances. The grandmother hypothesis is still 'only a hypothesis', and doesn't fully explain why humans, along with orcas, are so unusual in this respect, but it does remind us of the vital importance of older women to the health and survival of our species. Of course, older women have a value far beyond that of 'grandmothering', but our role as pod leaders, nurturers and repositories of wisdom is nevertheless an important one.

Who Wants to Live Forever?

Orca females outlive their male counterparts by about twenty or thirty years. Human females outlive their male counterparts by on average about five to ten years, depending on the country. In the UK, women live to on average 82.9 years, while men shuffle off at 79; in Australia and New Zealand, we live to 85.3 to their 81.2; in the US, it's 74.5 for men and 80.2 for the girls. This gap is repeated globally and without exception. And out of those people who live to the ripe old age of 100, women outnumber men by as many as nine to one. Why? Well, there's war, of course, and lifestyle factors like smoking, drinking excessive alcohol and hard manual labour, plus risk-taking behaviour, all of which tend to be more prevalent in men. But that doesn't explain everything. It's a myth, by the way, that the human lifespan has got increasingly longer – it's true that *life expectancy* was a lot lower in the nineteenth century – for example, because of infant mortality, disease and poverty – but it's important to distinguish this from *maximum lifespan*. In humans, lifespan has remained around 'three score years and ten' – with some making it into their nineties, just as we do today – since Roman times and probably before. A hundred or more years ago, life expectancy in both males and females was low, but if you managed to hang on until fifty or sixty and cheat death in childhood, childbirth or via the odd cholera epidemic, you could easily live, as most people globally still do today, to your mid-seventies. That extra decade or so beyond 75 that many of us now enjoy is likely to be thanks to better healthcare in our final years.[14] And, as far as we know, throughout history females have had the survival advantage over males.[15] Today, we die at lower rates than men from virtually all causes of death with the sole exception of Alzheimer's disease, to which we are particularly prone. It's still not fully understood why twice as many people with Alzheimer's are female – it used to be thought that it was simply because of women's longevity that we were more likely to get it. Now researchers are looking deeper and exploring other angles, including a link to oestrogen depletion, with some evidence to support the use of HRT, although more research is needed.[16] Lisa Mosconi, neuroscientist and author of *The Menopause Brain*, emphasises the role of a Mediterranean diet in Alzheimer's prevention, in particular the consumption of foods rich in phytoestrogens, such as flax and sesame seeds, soybeans, legumes, and a number of fruits and vegetables.

Our other Achilles heel, as females, are autoimmune disorders such as lupus and multiple sclerosis – around 80 per cent of those suffering from such disease are female. But this, according to Sharon Moalem, author of *The Better Half: On the Genetic Superiority of Women*, is because of our double helping of X chromosomes, which, while it can make our immune system prone to attack itself, for the most part works in our favour, making our immune system more powerful than men's. In genetics, Moalem says, the X chromosome 'has been mainly studied in terms of its negative health implications', while there has always been 'an incessant buzz' for the male Y chromosome, because, Moalem wryly suggests, 'most of the people who were speaking breathlessly about the Y had one as well'.

The science of chromosomes is another story of sexism – it was a woman, Nettie Stevens, who first observed the existence of XX and XY and their influence on development, but as is often the case, it was a man, Edmund Beecher Wilson, who took the credit. He apparently had access to her research results before they were published, and then used his influence to rush through his own paper on the subject before hers.[17] Once chromosomes then began to be studied, it was thought that females only made use of one of their X chromosomes, and that the other was 'switched off' early in our development – a pretty random thing to happen, when you think about it, but it does neatly position men as having an X *and* 'something extra' that women simply lack – that magical Y. One example of this bias is that medical students have long been taught that it's the X chromosome that's to blame for colour blindness, and also that women are much less likely to be colour-blind. What's left out of the story is that women are *more* likely to be able to perceive much more diversity of colour than men (ever picked out paint schemes with a male partner and found he's not got much of an opinion on whether you should go for 'Pewter' or 'Slate'?). 'At their genetic best,' says Moalem, 'men can only aspire to have normal colour vision.' Women, on the other hand, are not only likely to see much more variation, but may even have tetrachromatic vision – the ability to see 100 million colours instead of the usual 1 million. This is all because we have not one but two X chromosomes with two versions of the same genes, one compensating if the other has problems discerning colour.

Vision is far from the only area in which the extra X gives women an advantage. Rather than being dormant or inactive, our second X compensates and provides back-up to us consistently in times of need. Although in each female cell there is a dominant X chromosome, the other X is still active and accessible – giving us a genetic diversity that is lacking in males. From around twenty weeks of pregnancy to the very end of life, women have the survival advantage – females are less likely to be stillborn,[18] and less likely to be born prematurely,[19] but more likely to survive if they are.[20] Women are less likely to get non-sex-specific cancers but more likely to survive them,[21] better able to survive traumatic injury and more likely to survive extreme situations such as outbreaks of contagious disease, and they also do better in times of famine.[22] Researchers who looked at a variety of extreme humanitarian crises – from the Irish potato famine, to historic measles epidemics in Iceland, to plantation slavery in Trinidad – found that, across the board, women were more likely to survive than men. In the Covid pandemic, the spotlight was shone on this issue, because men were significantly more likely to die – in the first two months of the pandemic in England, for example, men were 30 per cent more likely to die.[23] In Spain, the virus had killed twice as many men as women by March 2020.[24] Moalem suggests this is again down to the second X. 'The X isn't just some random chromosome,' he explained in an interview for PBS news show *Amanpour & Co.* in April 2020.[25] 'It's actually very rich in genes that are related to the immune system. One gene specifically, TLR7, is a gene that recognises single-stranded RNA viruses, just like the coronavirus. So, practically speaking, what this means, in [the female] body, you have two immune cells that are using two different TLR7 genes to recognise the virus. So you have a big advantage there, because not only can you recognise it, you can then have on the other X a better gene to kill it. On the other hand, all my immune cells are using the exact same X. So I just have to hope that I have an X that's good enough not just to recognise the virus, but to kill it as well.'

Nevertheless, She Persisted

There are other theories about women's longevity. One is connected to both the second half of the menstrual cycle and pregnancy, times when researchers propose that oestrogen provokes cardiovascular changes, increasing cardiac output by as much as 20 per cent. This effect, which they have named the 'jogging female heart' could offer health benefits similar to the effects of exercise.[26] Other research suggests that oestrogen could also be acting as an antioxidant, mopping up the chemicals that cause stress – in animal experiments, females with their ovaries removed will not repair molecular damage as effectively.[27] The removal of the testes, however, has been shown to have the opposite effect in both animals and people: a study of eunuchs in the nineteenth-century court of the Chosun Dynasty of Korea found that these men, who'd had their testicles removed before puberty, lived to around seventy when other men of the court only made it to fifty.[28] Whether the eunuchs felt this trade-off was worthwhile is a whole other question.

How long a woman lives is also related to her reproductive history. Researchers who have looked at women who live to 100 or more have found that they were four times more likely to have had children in their forties than women who survived only to age 73.[29] Similarly, women who give birth to their first child earlier in life have been found to live shorter lives, most likely due to the socioeconomic factors that unfortunately go with early maternity.[30] Those who have children have been shown to live longer than those who don't, and this goes for fathers as well as mothers, and adoptive parents, too.[31] The number of children we have is also said to matter, with the sweet spot apparently being two or three, with gaps of two to three years between each (that's me – kerching!). Researchers are also looking at the relationship between childbirth and the brain and finding that women who have given birth have 'younger-looking brains' even in middle age.[32] The outliers to all of this are, of course, nuns, who are notorious for calmly reaching their centenary – there are apparently more nuns over ninety than under sixty. Nuns are thought to be fairly unique, however, not in their childlessness but in their sense of meaning and purpose, and their community-based lifestyle, supported by a tight-knit group of women.[33] Clearly, all kinds of women live to and beyond 100, some nuns, some mothers of many. The world's oldest recorded living human was a French woman called Jeanne Calment, who died in 1997 aged 122 years 164 days, and she had only one child at the age of 23. She clearly had a positive mindset – there are reports of practices such as daily expressions of gratitude (through prayer), regular fruit salads and up to a kilo a week of chocolate, and a reluctance to use either central heating or medicines. She gave up smoking at the age of 117. In 1969, age 94, she struck a deal under French law with her notary, a man named Raffray, to sell her apartment. Using a system called *en viager*, Raffray was to pay a monthly amount of 2,500 francs until taking ownership of the property on her death, which, since she was 94, he presumably wagered would not be too far off. Instead, Calment outlived him, and having shelled out each month for three decades, he died in 1995 having paid her nearly twice the value of her flat and never got the keys. 'In life, one sometimes makes bad deals,' she apparently said.[34] Some have even claimed Calment was a fraud, but her blood samples are yet to be studied and this has never been proven; in the meantime, she certainly fits the longevity profile of feisty and sharp: 'I've only got one wrinkle, and I'm sitting on it,' she famously said.

For the 'weaker sex', we women sure are tough. Women are now proving themselves to be every bit as good as men at extreme endurance sports such as ultrarunning and ultracycling.[35] I asked the ultrarunner and mum of three Sophie Power, whose image went viral after she was photographed breastfeeding her 3-month-old baby during the 106-mile Ultra-Trail du Mont-Blanc, whether she thought there was something about not just the female body, but the female psyche that was built to just keep going, the harder it got – something I know I've personally experienced in childbirth, if not in mountain running. 'Motherhood gives us a special set of superpowers in endurance racing,' she told me. 'We are well practised at sleep deprivation and the mental challenge of monotony. I race around a 400-metre track for twenty-four hours and it's just like my toddler asking me the same question again and again. Most of us have a birth experience that was more painful than anything we're likely to encounter on a race. In the late stages of pregnancy, we are in a state of constant discomfort, just like endurance racing, so we've had months of practice. We're also used to constantly looking after – often multiple – others. When I race it's easy as I only have to look after myself for once! So much of endurance racing is assessing how I feel, what I need, and solving problems that arise. I'm just doing it for myself rather than my three kids. Finally, as mothers, we've fought harder to be on those start lines than men. We have juggled family and work with training. For extreme events we have also fought against societal expectations of what women should and can do. When the going gets tough and quitting comes to mind, we can more easily jump another hurdle. Because we have already jumped so many hurdles to get on that start line and we may not get another chance to finish.' This is one part of female socialisation that is less talked about, and that you don't have to be a mother to experience – being female teaches you to be strong and to persist. As Olympic marathon runner Mara Yamauchi says, 'Female athletes, whether they are mothers or not, are tough and resilient. Women keep the world going through mountains of unpaid work and the lion's share of domestic duties and caring. Yet female athletes still find the time and energy to train and compete, despite numerous barriers.'

In a world in which, like Ginger Rogers, we have to do everything that Fred does, except backwards and in heels, women learn about endurance. Through the matriflux and its constant cycle of descent and return, like Inanna we learn how to persevere and endure. Could this mindset be at play, too, in our longevity, as we literally keep going longer and further than our male counterparts through life itself? The truth is, we just don't know the answers, although there does seem to be a connection between mindset and longevity. Much is made of the Japanese island of Okinawa, which famously has the highest ratio of centenarians and supercentenarians (people who live to 110) in the world, almost all of whom are women. Alongside a diet rich in plants and fresh, unprocessed food, the Okinawans have a mindset focus known as *ikigai*, which translates as 'life purpose' or 'why I wake up in the morning', and a built-in community-support network called *moai*, in which small groups of friends support each other for life. Okinawa is one of the world's five Blue Zones® – regions of the world identified by author Daniel Buettner and *National Geographic* as having exceptional longevity. All Blue Zones share the same lifestyle habits, named by Buettner as the 'Power 9', five of which concern mindset – a sense of purpose, taking time to reflect or de-stress, belonging (often to a faith-based community), strong social support networks (like *moai*) and an ethos of putting loved ones first. In Okinawa, this is epitomised by the saying, 'Live far enough away from your family so you aren't running into them every day, but close enough to take them a warm bowl of soup, on foot.' These values of caretaking and interconnectedness are often missing from our modern world, but it's perhaps worth mentioning that these are matriarchal values. As Dr Heide Göttner-Abendroth, feminist and expert in matriarchy, explains, 'Matriarchies are based on maternal values: care-taking, nurturing, motherliness, which holds for everybody: for mothers and those who are not mothers, for women and men alike.'[36] Post-menopause, bringing some of these values back into our lives could benefit others, and help us to live longer, too.

Anyone for a Sandwich?

It's unfortunate that any talk of creating a world more modelled on maternal values of care and nurture has to be accompanied by a caveat – it should not keep falling to women to pick up the slack. Post-menopausal women in their fifties and beyond may feel this acutely – they have been called the 'sandwich generation', responsible not just for the care and feeding of their teenage children, but also for their elderly parents as well. With people having babies later in life and then living longer, too, this sandwiching can even extend past our fifties into 'double sandwiches', in which four generations may be alive at once and find themselves working out structures of care that often place the greatest burden on the grandparents, who find themselves in their sixties, caring for their own parents who may be in their nineties, and at the same time offering much-needed childcare for their young grandchildren.

Those making up the bread in these many-layered sandwiches are almost always women.[37] 'Caring', which usually involves cooking and cleaning, as well as taking time to be with another person to talk, read or just be in their company, is, in spite of the feminist advances of recent decades, still thought of as 'women's work'. Some would argue that it's precisely because it's thought of as 'women's work' that it's so undervalued; perhaps it's not the specific nature of the work that we are undervaluing, but 'caring' itself, which does not hold much importance in a capitalist patriarchy. Caring professions are therefore paid less, but in particular if they are female dominated – for example, toilet cleaners get less than bin collectors, and a starting salary for a nurse is less than that of a paramedic.[38] So, if you scratch the surface, it's not just caring that we undervalue, it's women themselves. Caring is seen as 'feminine' and therefore both unimportant and ripe for exploitation.

Clearly there are huge issues with the gender pay gap, which affects post-menopausal women the most, but these are beyond the scope of this book.[39] There's also a difference between poorly paid care work and the 'care work' that women do for their children, parents and extended families. Some of this can be emotionally complex: caring for a terminally ill spouse is a different experience from caring for an ungrateful or unkind parent, and a sick child is different again. Caring for the people we love involves a mix of emotions, but it can also be fulfilling. I have to admit that, personally, I do really enjoy the sense of being needed by my children, and I don't think there are many areas of my life that make me as happy – truly, deeply happy, not just the kind of happiness I experience with my first beach cocktail – than just 'being there' for them. I don't always feel this way on a day-to-day basis, though, and it can tip over into frustration when I feel I don't get any time for myself, or when I feel taken for granted. In the worst of times, caring can feel like thankless drudgery. This is the rub, I think – it's when it feels like an injustice, as though it's a task that's falling to us specifically because we are female, that it starts to grate. So perhaps, rather than denigrate care work itself and try to find ways to delegate it (often to other, low-waged women), we need to think about a new social model, in which, instead of family care work being framed as drudgery, a way of enslaving women and capitalising on their unselfish ability to put others first and their own dreams to the side, we instead look at ways to make it part of everyone's daily lives, male or female. Societies with care and nurture at their heart have a better quality of life and live longer, too – so it would be to everyone's advantage to create social structures and government policy to support this ideal.

Elder, Not Elderly

'Men don't age better than women,
they're just allowed to age.'

CARRIE FISHER

Being an old woman in the world is perhaps more complex now than ever. Slammed between two poles of ageing naturally and the widely available options of fillers and lifts; told to be our 'authentic selves' but offered filters on social media that will instantly take years off our age – we are, as usual, damned if we do and damned if we don't. The impossible goal is to look like we did at 35 without having any 'tweakments', and to age naturally without actually looking any older. Tabloid headlines about female celebrities over sixty regularly describe them as 'unrecognisable', as if it's a shock that they don't still look like they did thirty years ago. After the 2023 Grammy Awards, Piers Morgan tweeted a picture of the 64-year-old Madonna captioned, 'I thought Halloween was in October?' In an Instagram post responding to the furore, Madonna slammed 'the glare of ageism and misogyny that permeates the world we live in . . . A world that refuses to celebrate women past the age of 45 and feels the need to punish her if she continues to be strong-willed, hard-working and adventurous.' Madonna, like many female celebrities, has chosen to have work done to her face, and is slated anyway, presumably because it doesn't 'look natural', but women who genuinely 'look natural', such as Mary Beard, are subject to regular abuse and references to their personal appearance: 'Throughout many periods of history in the West there has been a real worry about what you do with women who are past their childbearing years. As I can confirm, women with long grey hair can make people anxious,' Beard said, adding, 'I have frequently been called a witch on Twitter.'[40]

Can we reframe this cronehood? The word 'crone' is said to come from the word 'carrion', as in 'decaying flesh', which sounds like a difficult concept to put a positive spin on, even for me. However, the Jungian analyst and author of *Women Who Run with the Wolves* Clarissa Pinkola Estés has suggested the word has links to 'crown' or '*la corona*', one who has reached a great level of insight: queen. Others have suggested that 'hag', rather than deriving from the old English for 'harpy' or 'witch', instead comes from 'hagio', meaning holy or divine. A bit of digging takes you to the Old Norse 'hagi', meaning 'sacred grove', and the Shakespearean words 'hagged', meaning 'bewitched', and 'haggard', meaning 'untamed'. And the word 'witch' is said to derive from the Old English 'wicca' and 'wicce', meaning male and female witch, but this, too, is debated, with some suggesting instead that the word comes from 'wit', meaning wisdom, knowledge and understanding. In France, women have set up a female-only communal retirement complex, reclaiming pride in their hag phase by the name they have chosen: 'Baba Yaga's House'. The founder of the commune, Thérèse Clerc, said, 'To live long is a good thing but to age well is better.' Remember Frigg and Freya from Chapter 2 (see page 45), the goddesses after whom Friday is named? They were the Viking shamans known as *völvas*, females with magic wands, the ability to shape-shift into falcons and to manipulate fate itself. From Sylvia Keepers via Jane Hardwicke Collings, we have our new word maga, the woman between mother and crone – the wise woman, the enchantress, the autumn woman – who is standing right in her power and harvesting the fruits of her labours. Some feel the word 'elder' is also ripe for reclaiming, along with the idea that older people should be respected and revered, rather than sidelined and labelled as 'elderly'. It is for each woman to decide what she feels herself to be and how she describes herself, but the words we choose matter and indicate our feelings and intentions.

Witches, hags, crones, *völvas*, Baba Yagas – all of these old women figures are simultaneously feared and revered. While writing this chapter I was sitting in a completely unrelated meeting with my 15-year-old daughter and a woman in her sixties. As the older woman was speaking, I suddenly realised

I was automatically having critical thoughts when I looked at her face, and I sat, observing myself for a moment. 'Her hair is so rough and wiry . . . She has double chins . . . I can see all the pores round her nose and the veins in her cheeks . . . Her complexion is rough . . .' and so on. I had caught myself red-handed, almost on auto-pilot, judging this woman and her very visible signs of age. I stopped myself, and looked again, and made myself consciously look for the beauty instead. I noticed the small touches she had made to her appearance: different-coloured liners above and below her eyes, an interesting glasses chain, silver and gold and beads adorning her that I imagined all had their own stories. Her posture, like her hair, which I had previously judged so harshly, was jaunty and unapologetic, and her body had the solidity that only comes from several decades of moving and cooking and eating and living – a true 'goddess body', taking up space. As she talked I glanced across at my daughter, and noticed her, too. Fifteen, her body slender, her skin pale, smooth and elastic, in complete contrast to the older woman's expansive frame and wide, ruddy face. Where had I learned to prize one over the other? I think we all know the answer to that. We hand it down, from generation to generation, mother to daughter, our own internalised self-loathing and ageism and misogyny and fear, all projected outwards where it becomes, 'Such awful hair!' or, 'What *IS* she wearing?' We teach it to our daughters every time we criticise our own reflection, and as soon as we realise this, we can immediately take steps to break this cycle. Change starts with noticing what needs to change.

I looked from one to the other, my daughter, and the older woman, and, of course, me . . . sitting between them both, the halfway point. Maiden. Mother. Maga. The three of us, each just a different iteration of the same; each on our journey through the matriflux; each with our power manifesting in different ways; each the other's guide, sister, ally.

Thoughts on Reaching the End

'Rage, rage against the dying of the light.'

DYLAN THOMAS, *Do Not Go Gentle into That Good Night*

'Every gambler knows
That the secret to survivin'
Is knowin' what to throw away
And knowin' what to keep
'Cause every hand's a winner
And every hand's a loser
And the best that you can hope for
Is to die in your sleep.'

KENNY ROGERS, *The Gambler*

As I've gone through the process of researching and writing this book, my social-media posts and Google searches have completely confuzzled the algorithms. I've had cookies dropped on me on a huge range of topics all the way through from puberty to death, with advertisers scrambling over themselves to sell me tampons . . . no, wait . . . maternity wear . . . no, hang on . . . baby wipes . . . just a second . . . how about a supplement for your hot flushes . . .? A retirement villa . . .? A coffin . . .? I like to visualise a large room, somewhere in Silicon Valley, filled with servers and tangles of wires, fizzing and sparking away as it tries to work out precisely what product to flog me until it finally combusts in a cartoon fireball.

For each chapter, a life stage, and for each life stage, a marketing opportunity. I don't know much about business, but I do know that if you want to sell people something it's a good idea to think about a problem they have and then position your product as a solution to it. And if they don't have a problem, don't worry – the very existence of your product will persuade them that they do. Women, who drive consumer spending, are the sex that advertisers most wish to reach. And, boy, do they have a lot of problems! They can't get through pregnancy without a U-shaped body pillow in organic cotton stuffed with lavender from the fields of Provence; they'll be terrible mothers if they don't get that educational set of rustic yet splinter-free stacking logs; they absolutely can't go through menopause without a handbag-sized cryospheric hot-and-cold roller ball in life-enhancing purple. The matriflux is so ripe for exploitation that if I don't register the word matriflux as a trademark before this book comes out, there'll be a cycle-tracking bracelet with Swarovski-crystal accents named after it by Christmas.

The stories we tell about life in the female body, these body myths, don't only serve to sell us more stuff, it's worse than that. They undermine us. They chip, chip, chip at our confidence and convince us to spend our lives on the back foot, our voices quietened, our postures made smaller, our opening words always an apology. 'Sorry but I really think . . .', 'Sorry would you mind if I just . . .' all of these turns of phrase have their roots in the body myths that remind us of our inferiority and inadequacy. Have you ever had a friend or relative or partner who constantly picked faults, criticised you or made endless negative comments? After a while, you start to believe them, don't you, and it becomes harder and harder to stand tall. I hope this book is the new friend who comes along and tells you you're brilliant, just when you need to hear it most. Often, all it takes is just one friend, or one book, to tip you over into a new way of thinking, and then there's no going back to the old, destructive ways.

When my dad was in his eighties he used to tell me that all the sugar was at the bottom of the cup, and I won't know if that's really true until I get there, I guess. Maybe it's not saccharine at all but quite awful knowing you're at the end of your life and might not wake up tomorrow morning, or maybe it's a mix. Certainly, coming to the end of the process of writing a book is not emotionally straightforward; I am not the only writer to report that, rather than a sense of achievement and contentment, typing the words 'The End' can be deeply anxiety provoking. Did I fill those pages to the best of my abilities? Could I have tried harder? Will any gaps and mistakes be as vivid to other people as they are to me? And, now that I have laid this imperfect work out on the table for everyone to see, how will I be judged? There's nothing like an ending to bring on a bit of an existential crisis, followed by a deep sigh of resignation and the desire to say something vaguely meaningful about sweetened cups of tea.

Much of the focus of this book has been on the reality of

a lifetime in a physical body, which on the one hand can make you feel vividly alive, but on the other put you firmly in touch with the reality of your mortality, and your inevitable deterioration and demise. Throughout history and culture humans have found creative ways to express the concept of '*memento mori*', or 'remember that you die', somehow realising that pictures of skulls emblazoned with doom-laden slogans have the paradoxical effect of giving us a new lease of life. Women's bodies are one great big living, breathing *memento mori*; they leave blood on the sheets as proof. I have never felt so alive as the days I birthed my three children into the world, with death so close I could almost touch it. And giving birth took away some of my fear of death. I can remember thinking, in the throes of each labour, *Oh, so this is what death will be like. When it comes, turns out I won't really mind that much, because just like this, I will be so utterly focused on what's happening in my body. This is what they mean when they say, 'Be here now.'* And then I got on with the business of getting a new human out into the world and watching them take their first-ever breath.

The *memento mori* is not currently fashionable in Western culture. We don't want to wear little charms filled with the hair of deceased loved ones, or have their bodies laid out in our front parlour. Quite the opposite: our relationship with the body has become one of complete denial of its mammalian and impermanent nature. All of us, but women in particular, are supposed to cheat the Reaper himself with a combination of dieting and exercise fads, supplements, pills, age-defying face creams and clock-denying tweakments. The body has become something we 'own', like a car, which can not only be maintained but also upgraded and enhanced; new parts added, unwanted parts removed. Researching and writing this book in a linear way, from cradle to grave, has been a *memento mori* of sorts, but the exploration of the matriflux has also been a reminder of the cyclical, never-ending nature of life and death. Each month, a menstruating woman flows through different states, her progress mirroring the progress of the day through dawn, morning, midday, afternoon, dusk, sunset, darkness, sunrise, and round, and round. This in turn mirrors the seasons: spring, summer, autumn, winter and then back again to spring. And these seasons mirror the cycle of life itself, as she progresses through times of new shoots, bloom, fade, decay. When she reaches menopause, this is an end of sorts, but also a return to the beginning, as oestrogen and progesterone go back to pre-puberty levels, and she may simultaneously find herself reconnecting with the hopes, dreams and passions of her childhood self. Through her creative powers, even as she fades into the winter of her life, and dies, she will live on through the people and the projects she has brought forth into the world during her fertile times. Birth, life, death, rebirth: the matriflux endlessly cycles.

Reconnecting with the power of the female body brings us back into deep connection with the very nature of being alive. This book has asked you not just to contemplate that power, but to reframe the idea of power itself from one of dominance and control to one of fertility and creativity. In a world that insists that anyone who says there is something unique or special about being female is either trying to chain women to their reproductive abilities, suggest that they are in some way limited or inferior, or even act as a kind of gatekeeper to womanhood itself, the meaning of this bears repeating: the female body is in possession of a creative power that can be used in a multitude of ways, only one of which is reproduction. Women are discouraged from any focus on this unique power, often being taught that any discussion of it is bad for feminism. Added to this, generation after generation of women have also been taught that their bodies are a source of pain, inconvenience, weakness and shame. Isn't it time for us to reframe and reclaim these ideas, and start to train ourselves – and our daughters – to think about being female as a privilege? After all, if we are born female, we will die female. Should we spend the time in between those two fixed dates cursing our bodies, or can we change the way we talk about them, and the way we feel about them, for good?

Each time I have shared even the smallest hint of some of the science I've included in this book on social media, women have devoured it with a wild appetite. On Mother's Day in March 2023, for example, I shared a Twitter thread about foetal microchimerism (described in Chapter 3, page 98), and the way in which cells from our babies, even those we did not carry to term, may still be in our bodies decades later, and that cells from our own mothers may also still be with us. The response can only be described as a huge outpouring of bittersweetness; happiness and incredulity that this was not just a metaphor, but a physical reality, and grief for the mothers and children that people had lost but were now overwhelmed to think were still with them physically in some way. Thousands of women liked, shared and commented. For me, this reinforced the point of this book – women's bodies are truly amazing and leaning in to the fine details about how they work can really change the way we feel about and experience these bodies in profound and moving ways.

For me, writing this book has changed the way I feel about my own body. It has shone a spotlight on each phase of life and, as I've travelled through the chapters, forced me to confront my own negative feelings and expectations, question my automatic thoughts that stem from generations of damage, and keep asking instead, 'What's good about this?' What's good about being female? Looking in the mirror as I move into my fifties, I know there is work for me to do on embracing the person I am now as my face and body changes and ages. Every decade of life in the matriflux brings these inevitable transformations. But the key, I believe, is in repeatedly shifting the focus away from how we look, and onto what our bodies have done, and can still do. Rather than, 'I am beautiful, no matter what they say,' I need to sing, 'I am powerful, no matter what they say.' I am strong. This new kind of body positivity, with its focus on inner power rather than outer appearance, is what I hope is one of the key takeaways of this book. Superficial, cosmetic changes will not bring us the solutions we seek. We have to come back to the body itself, become curious about it and fascinated with it, as if it is a new country. And each time we find a story of shame or inadequacy, we need to remember to wipe away those cultural, historical and often patriarchal layers to find what is beneath. There will always be a story of power hidden there under each body myth.

We have to say, 'No more shame.' We have to replace those shameful myths with the facts that science now offers us. We have to carve out a new world that works for us, as cyclical beings, refusing to accept any longer that our biology is a sign of our weakness and must therefore not be mentioned. And we have to come back to the body, to our real, active, purposeful bodies, as they are today, and love them for all their imperfection and fragility. The female body is brilliant. Life in it is brilliant. Eventually, everything ends. *Memento mori.*

Acknowledgements

With thanks to my agent Jane at Graham Maw Christie, and to Lisa Milton, Danielle Pender and the team at HQ Stories for their care and expertise in bringing this book to publication. Also thanks and love to my three children for their inspiration and encouragement.

Endnotes

Chapter 1

1. Mobius, M. M. and Rosenblat, T. S. (2006). 'Why beauty matters', *The American Economic Review*, 96(1), pp. 222–235. doi: 10.1257/000282806776157515.
2. Efran, M. G. (1974). 'The effect of physical appearance on the judgment of guilt, interpersonal attraction, and severity of recommended punishment in a simulated jury task', *Journal of Research in Personality*, 8(1), pp. 45–54. doi: 10.1016/0092-6566(74)90044-0.
3. Mulvey, L. (1975). 'Visual Pleasure and Narrative Cinema', *Screen*, 16(3), pp. 6–18. doi: 10.1093/screen/16.3.6.
4. Atwood, M. (2020). *The Robber Bride*. London: Little, Brown Book Group.
5. UK Parliament (2020). *Body Image Survey Results, Women and Equalities Committee*, 23 September. Available at: https://publications.parliament.uk/pa/cm5801/cmselect/cmwomeq/805/80502.htm
6. Dreisbach, S. (2011). 'Shocking bodyimage news: 97% of women will be cruel to their bodies today', *Glamour*, 3 February. Available at: https://www.glamour.com/story/

shocking-body-image-news-97-percent-of-women-will-be-cruel-to-their-bodies-today

7. UCL (2026). '1.6 million UK adults used weight loss drugs in past year', *UCL News*, 8 January. Available at: https://www.ucl.ac.uk/news/2026/jan/16-million-uk-adults-used-weight-loss-drugs-past-year
8. Luthra, S. (2023). 'Weightloss drugs like Ozempic are more likely to interest women than men, poll finds', *The 19th*, 4 August. Available at: https://19thnews.org/2023/08/weight-loss-drugs-ozempic-women-poll
9. MacDonnell, C. (2025). '"A 360 turn": concern as fashion shows feature fewer plussize models', *The Guardian*, 17 October. Available at: https://www.theguardian.com/fashion/2025/oct/17/fashion-shows-fewer-plus-size-models-vogue-business
10. Davies, H. (2025). 'Lizzo's "No" to Ozempic: Plussize women are being "erased" by Ozempic "boom", claims "proud big girl" pop star Lizzo', *The Sun*, 24 November. Available at: https://www.thesun.co.uk/tvandshowbiz/37426284/lizzo-plus-size-women-erased-ozempic/
11. Wells, L. (2025). 'Plastic Surgery Comes for the Waist', *The New York Times*, 12 October. Available at: https://www.nytimes.com/2025/10/12/style/plastic-surgery-waist-reduction.html
12. Ceurstemont, S. (2026). 'We're finally learning the true sideeffects of weightloss drugs', *BBC Science Focus*, 21 January. Available at: https://www.sciencefocus.com/the-human-body/dark-side-of-weight-loss-drugs

13. West, S., Scragg, J., Aveyard, P., Oke, J. L., Willis, L., Haffner, S. J. P., Knight, H., Wang, D., Morrow, S., Heath, L., Jebb, S. A. and Koutoukidis, D. A. (2026). 'Weight regain after cessation of medication for weight management: systematic review and metaanalysis', BMJ, 392. doi: 10.1136/bmj-2025-085304.
14. Pharmaceutical Executive (2023). *Global Obesity Drug Sales Expected to Hit $44 Billion by 2030*, 1 June. Available at: https://www.pharmexec.com/view/global-obesity-drug-sales-expected-to-hit-44-billion-by-2030
15. Pulter, H. (no date). 'Made When I Was Not Well', in Eardley, A. and Butler, D. (eds.) *The Pulter Project: Poetical Works of Lady Hester Pulter*. Available at: https://pulterproject.northwestern.edu/poems/ee/made-when-i-was-not-well/
16. Verified Market Research (2026). 'Cosmetic surgery market size worth $64.88 billion, globally, by 2028 at 3.54% CAGR', *PR Newswire*, 16 November. Available at: https://www.prnewswire.com/news-releases/cosmetic-surgery-market-size-worth--64-88-billion-globally-by-2028-at-3-54-cagr-verified-market-research-301425313.html
17. Grand View Research (2022). 'Cosmetic Surgery and Procedure Market Size Worth $145.7 Billion by 2030', *Bloomberg*, 15 March. Available at: https://www.bloomberg.com/press-releases/2022-03-15/cosmetic-surgery-and-procedure-market-size-worth-145-7-billion-by-2030-grand-view-research-inc

18. NHS (2024). *Tummy tuck (abdominoplasty)*, 7 May. Available at: https://www.nhs.uk/conditions/cosmetic-procedures/tummy-tuck/
19. NHS (2023). *Breast enlargement (implants)*, 22 September. Available at: https://www.nhs.uk/conditions/cosmetic-procedures/breast-enlargement/
20. NHS (2023). *Labiaplasty*, 27 September. Available at: https://www.nhs.uk/tests-and-treatments/cosmetic-procedures/cosmetic-surgery/labiaplasty/
21. Kalampalikis, A. and Michala, L. (2021). 'Cosmetic labiaplasty on minors: a review of current trends and evidence', *International Journal of Impotence Research*, 35(3), pp. 192–195. doi: 10.1038/s41443-021-00480-1.
22. Boddy, J. (2016). 'The normal and the aberrant in female genital cutting', *HAU: Journal of Ethnographic Theory*, 6(2), 41–69. https://doi.org/10.14318/hau6.2.008.
23. Kassel, G. (2020). 'Everything you need to know about labiaplasty', *Healthline*, 29 January. Available at: https://www.healthline.com/health/labiaplasty
24. O'Regan, K. (2013). 'Labiaplasty, Part I', *Guernica*, 16 January. Available at: https://www.guernicamag.com/kirsten-oregan-labiaplasty-part-i/
25. South Coast Urogynecology (no date). *Aesthetic vaginal surgery*. Available at: https://urogyn.org/services/aesthetic-vaginal-surgery/
26. Forster, K. (2017). 'Labiaplasty: Vaginal surgery "world's fastestgrowing cosmetic procedure", say plastic surgeons', *The Independent*, 12 July. Available at: https://www.independent.co.uk/news/health/

labiaplasty-vagina-surgery-cosmetic-procedure-plastic-study-international-society-aesthetic-plastic-surgeons-usa-a7837181.html

27. George, R. (2018). 'The vagina is selfcleaning – so why does the "feminine hygiene" industry exist?', *The Guardian*, 4 September. Available at: https://www.theguardian.com/society/2018/sep/04/the-vagina-is-self-cleaning-so-why-does-the-feminine-hygiene-industry-exist
28. Mental Health Foundation (no date). *Men and women: statistics*. Available at: https://www.mentalhealth.org.uk/explore-mental-health/statistics/men-women-statistics
29. Freeman, H. (2018). 'I had anorexia – but not because I wanted to look like a fashion model', *The Guardian*, 19 March. Available at: https://www.theguardian.com/commentisfree/2015/mar/19/eating-model-french-skinny-anorexia
30. Bindel, J. (7 January 2023). 'Haley Freeman: Best selling author, columnist and feature writer for the Sunday Times', *Julie Bindel's writing and podcasts*. Available at: https://juliebindel.substack.com/p/hadley-freeman-best-selling-author
31. NHS (2020). *Gender dysphoria*, 28 May. Available at: https://www.nhs.uk/conditions/gender-dysphoria/
32. Gentleman, A. (2022). '"An explosion": what is behind the rise in girls questioning their gender identity?', *The Guardian*, 24 November. Available at: https://www.theguardian.com/society/2022/nov/24/an-explosion-what-is-behind-the-rise-in-girls-questioning-their-gender-identity

33. UK Parliament (no date). *Written evidence submitted by Transgender Trend (MISS0046)*. Available at: https://committees.parliament.uk/writtenevidence/7947/html
34. Stein, J. (2022). 'Who is Monica Sjöö?', *FiLiA*, 22 August. Available at: https://www.filia.org.uk/latest-news/2022/8/10/who-is-monica-sj
35. The Sheela Na Gig Project (no date). *Buncton/Wiston*. Available at: https://sheelanagig.org/buncton/
36. Dwyer, B. (no date). 'Sheelanagigs and an "Aesthetics of Damage"', *Enclave Review*. Available at: http://enclavereview.org/sheela-na-gigs-and-an-aesthetics-of-damage/
37. Hitchcock, D. (no date). 'The Vulva in Stone Age Art', *Don's Maps*. Available at: https://donsmaps.com/vulvastoneage.html
38. SteinkopfFrank, H. (2021). 'What's up with all the lady parts in medieval prayer books?', *Messy Nessy Chic*, 2 July. Available at: https://www.messynessychic.com/2021/06/30/whats-up-with-all-the-lady-parts-in-medieval-prayer-books/
39. Pearson, E. A. (2002). 'Revealing and concealing: The persistence of vaginal iconography in medieval imagery. The mandorla, the vesica piscis, the rose, Sheelanagigs and the doubletailed mermaid', *uOttawa*. Available at: https://ruor.uottawa.ca/handle/10393/6133
40. Wood, C. (no date). 'Mother Mary and the Goddess', *Interfaith Mary*. Available at: https://www.interfaithmary.net/articles/mary-goddess
41. Blackledge. C. (2020). *Raising the Skirt: The Unsung Power of the Vagina*. London: Weidenfeld & Nicolson Ltd.

42. Walker, D. (2023). 'Police Scotland drop "ludicrous" probe into fake flasher protest at Holyrood', *Scottish Daily Express*, 13 January. Available at: https://www.scottishdailyexpress.co.uk/news/politics/police-scotland-drop-ludicrous-probe-28946411
43. Weiss, S. (2023). '"Our Bodies, Ourselves" taught women about sexuality and reproductive health', *Washington Post*, 21 May. Available at: https://www.washingtonpost.com/national/health-science/our-bodies-ourselves-taught-women-about-sexuality-and-reproductive-health/2011/09/22/gIQAdkV6IL_story.html
44. Walsh, K. (2024). 'Gillian Anderson wore a dress embroidered with vaginas at the Golden Globes, and we almost missed it', *Glamour UK*, 9 January. Available at: https://www.glamourmagazine.co.uk/article/gillian-anderson-dress-embroidered-vaginas-golden-globes-2024
45. Geddes, L. (2021). 'Most Britons cannot name all parts of the vulva, survey reveals', *The Guardian*, 30 May. Available at: https://www.theguardian.com/lifeandstyle/2021/may/30/most-britons-cannot-name-parts-vulva-survey
46. The Eve Appeal (2017). *Not Just Women's Troubles - #KnowYourBody this Gynae Month*, 31 August. Available at: https://eveappeal.org.uk/blog/not-just-womens-troubles/
47. Endometriosis UK (no date). *Endometriosis facts and figures*. Available at: https://www.endometriosis-uk.org/endometriosis-facts-and-figures#
48. Kwint, J. (2022). Women's Health: 'Why do women feel unheard?', *National Institute for Health and Care Research*. doi: 10.3310/nihrevidence_54676.

49. O'Connell, P. H. (2020). *Get Cliterate* [online video], TED Talks, 15 August. Available at: https://www.ted.com/talks/professor_helen_o_connell_get_cliterate
50. King, H. (2023). 'The clitoris – a brief history', *The Conversation*, 4 January. Available at: https://theconversation.com/the-clitoris-a-brief-history-196817
51. Wahlquist, C. (2020). 'The sole function of the clitoris is female orgasm. Is that why it's ignored by medical science?', *The Guardian*, 31 October. Available at: https://www.theguardian.com/lifeandstyle/2020/nov/01/the-sole-function-of-the-clitoris-is-female-orgasm-is-that-why-its-ignored-by-medical-science
52. Frederick, D. A., St John, H. K., Garcia, J. R. and Lloyd, E. A. (2017). 'Differences in orgasm frequency among gay, lesbian, bisexual, and heterosexual men and women in a U.S. national sample', *Archives of Sexual Behavior*, 47(1), pp. 273–288. doi: 10.1007/s10508-017-0939-z.
53. Kratochvíl, S. (1993). 'Multiple orgasms in women', *PubMed*, 1 December. Available at: https://pubmed.ncbi.nlm.nih.gov/8124735/
54. Mintz, L. (2022). 'To close the gap, we need to hold penetration and clitoral stimulation as equal', *Psychology Today*, 24 February. Available at: https://www.psychologytoday.com/gb/blog/stress-and-sex/201510/the-orgasm-gap-simple-truth-sexual-solutions
55. Morris, N. (2015). 'Women have more intense orgasms through masturbation than through sex', *Metro*, 4 October. Available at: https://metro.co.uk/2021/08/17/

women-have-more-intense-orgasms-through-masturbation-than-through-sex-15103514/

56. Klein, V. and Conley, T. D. (2021). 'The role of gendered entitlement in understanding inequality in the bedroom', *Social Psychological & Personality Science*, 13(6), pp. 1047–1057. doi: 10.1177/19485506211053564.
57. Afshari P., Houshyar Z., Javadifar N., Pourmotahari F., & Jorfi M. (25 November 2026). 'The Relationship Between Body Image and Sexual Function in Middle-Aged Women', *Electron Physician*, *8*(11), 3302-3308. https://doi.org/10.19082/3302.
58. Quinn-Nilas C., Benson L., Milhausen R. R., Buchholz A. C., & Goncalves M. (29 March 2016). 'The Relationship Between Body Image and Domains of Sexual Functioning Among Heterosexual, Emerging Adult Women', *Sexual Medicine*, *4*(3), 182-9. https://doi.org/10.1016/j.esxm.2016.02.004.
59. Ragosa, M. R. (no date). 'Strong & Beautiful: How weightlifting is improving the selfimage of women', *Invictus Fitness*. Available at: https://www.crossfitinvictus.com/blog/strong-beautiful-weightlifting-improving-self-image-women/
60. Gordon, B. R., McDowell, C. P., Hallgren, M., Meyer, J. D., Lyons, M. and Herring, M. P. (2018). 'Association of efficacy of resistance exercise training with depressive symptoms', *JAMA Psychiatry*, 75(6), p. 566. doi: 10.1001/jamapsychiatry.2018.0572.
61. Shaw, G. (2009). 'Women and weight training for osteoporosis', *WebMD*, 20 January. Available at: https://www.webmd.com/osteoporosis/features/weight-training

62. Westcott, W. L. (2012). 'Resistance training is medicine', *Current Sports Medicine Reports*, 11(4), pp. 209–216. doi: 10.1249/JSR.0b013e31825dabb8.
63. Harvard T. H. Chan School of Public Health (2022). *Evidence mounts on the benefits of strength training*, 17 March. Available at: https://www.hsph.harvard.edu/news/hsph-in-the-news/strength-training-time-benefits/

Chapter 2

1. McCoy, D. (no date). 'FRIGG', *Norse Mythology for Smart People*. Available at: https://norse-mythology.org/gods-and-creatures/the-aesir-gods-and-goddesses/frigg/
2. McCoy, D. (no date). 'Seldr', *Norse Mythology for Smart People*. Available at: https://norse-mythology.org/concepts/seidr/
3. King, H. (2013). 'Menotoxin – when menstruation can kill?', *Wonders & Marvels*, 10 September. Available at: https://www.wondersandmarvels.com/2013/09/menotoxin-when-menstruation-can-kill.html
4. Melchor, A. (2021). 'Posies, Poison, and Periods, early 1920s', *The Scientist Magazine*, 31 August. Available at: https://www.the-scientist.com/foundations/posies-poison-and-periods-early-1920s-69075
5. Ailsa (2021a). 'Menotoxins in a history of periods: impurity or superstition?', *Vulvani*, 11 October. Available at: https://www.vulvani.com/en/menotoxins-in-a-history-of-periods-impurity-or-superstition

6. Ailsa (2021b). 'Menotoxins in a history of periods: impurity or superstition?', *Vulvani*, 11 October. Available at: https://www.vulvani.com/en/menotoxins-in-a-history-of-periods-impurity-or-superstition
7. Bhartiya, A. & Indian Institute of Technology Roorkee (2013). 'Menstruation, religion and society', *International Journal of Social Science and Humanity*, 3(6), pp. 523–523. doi: 10.7763/IJSSH.2013.V3.296.
8. SikhiToTheMax (no date). *ANG 473 of Guru Granth Sahib Ji*. Available at: https://www.sikhitothemax.org/ang?ang=473
9. UNESCO (2014). *Puberty education & menstrual hygiene management*. Available at: https://unesdoc.unesco.org/ark:/48223/pf0000226792
10. Women News Network (2011). *Nepal banishment ritual for girls*, 20 March. Available at: https://womennewsnetwork.net/2011/03/20/nepal-banishment-ritual-girls/
11. ActionAid UK (2023). *Chhaupadi and menstruation taboos*, 31 January. Available at: https://www.actionaid.org.uk/our-work/period-poverty/chhaupadi-and-menstruation-taboos
12. Steinem, G. (2019). 'If men could menstruate', *Women's Reproductive Health*, 6(3), pp. 151–152. doi: 10.1080/23293691.2019.1619050.
13. BBC News (2017). *Bodyform advert replaces blue liquid with red 'blood'*, 18 October. Available at: https://www.bbc.co.uk/news/uk-41666280
14. Terlep, S. (2020). 'Kotex decides women's blood is red, not blue', *The Wall Street Journal*, 23 January. Available at: https://www.wsj.com/articles/kotex-decides-womens-blood-is-red-not-blue-11579800492

15. Mertens, M. (2015). 'Great moments in menstrual history', *The Cut*, 14 September. Available at: https://www.thecut.com/2015/09/great-moments-in-menstrual-history.html
16. Adams, R. (2010). 'Tampon-makers can't mention the V-word. Period', *The Guardian*, 17 March. Available at: https://www.theguardian.com/world/richard-adams-blog/2010/mar/16/tampon-vagina-kotex-advertising
17. Kaur, R. (2025). Available at: https://www.instagram.com/p/0ovWwJHA6f/
18. Grahn, J. (1993/2007). 'All blood is menstrual blood', *Metaformia*. Available at: http://www.metaformia.org/poetry/all-blood/
19. Braithwaite, J. (2022). 'Period survey results: Workplace stigma and most common symptoms', *Forth*, 14 September. Available at: https://www.forthwithlife.co.uk/blog/period-survey-workplace-stigma-symptoms/
20. Always (no date). *Breaking Period Stigma with New Report from Always®*. Available at: https://www.always.co.uk/en-gb/breaking-period-stigma/
21. Menstrual Hygiene Day (no date). *Always_WASH_United: Glocalities — Period Stigma Around the World Today 2021*. Available at: https://menstrualhygieneday.org/wp-content/uploads/2021/06/Always_WASH_United__Glocalities_Period_Stigma_Around_the_World_Today_2021.pdf
22. Clue (2021). *Menstrual euphemisms by language*, 14 April. Available at: https://helloclue.com/articles/culture/top-euphemisms-for-period-by-language
23. Briden, L. (2021). 'How to improve premenstrual mood symptoms (A summary of natural treatments)', *The Period*

Revolutionary, 11 December. Available at: https://www.larabriden.com/how-to-improve-premenstrual-mood-symptoms/

24. Hill, M. (no date). Available at: https://twitter.com/millihill/status/1595822154364354561
25. Hantsoo, L. & Epperson, C. N. (2015). 'Premenstrual Dysphoric Disorder: Epidemiology and treatment', *Current Psychiatry Reports*, 17(11). doi: 10.1007/s11920-015-0628-3.
26. University of North Carolina at Chapel Hill (1998). 'Severe PMS linked with physical, sexual abuse in childhood', *ScienceDaily*, 13 November. Available at: https://www.sciencedaily.com/releases/1998/11/981113082005.htm
27. Eisenlohr-Moul, T. (2019). 'Premenstrual Disorders: A primer and research agenda for psychologists', *PubMed Central*, 1 January. Available at: https://www.ncbi.nlm.nih.gov/pmc/articles/PMC7193982/#R25
28. Emma (2017). 'The gender wars of household chores: a feminist comic', *The Guardian*, 26 May. Available at: https://www.theguardian.com/world/2017/may/26/gender-wars-household-chores-comic
29. Gollenberg, A. L., Hediger, M. L., Mumford, S. L., Whitcomb, B. W., Hovey, K. M., Wactawski-Wende, J. & Schisterman, E. F. (2010). 'Perceived stress and severity of perimenstrual symptoms: the BioCycle Study', *Journal of Women's Health*, 19(5), pp. 959–967. doi: 10.1089/jwh.2009.1717.
30. Bertone-Johnson, E. R., Whitcomb, B. W., Missmer, S. A., Manson, J. E., Hankinson, S. E. & Rich-Edwards, J. W. (2014). 'Early life emotional, physical, and sexual abuse and

the development of premenstrual syndrome: a longitudinal study', *Journal of Women's Health*, 23(9), pp. 729–739. doi: 10.1089/jwh.2013.4674.

31. Koci, A. & Strickland, O. (2009). 'Relationship of adolescent physical and sexual abuse to perimenstrual symptoms (PMS) in adulthood', *Issues in Mental Health Nursing*, 28(1), pp. 75–87. doi: 10.1080/01612840600996281.
32. Pelz, M. & Chatterjee, R. (2023). 'Fasting, Hormones & Menopause: Why Women Need a Different Approach to Men' [Podcast], *Feel Better, Live More with Dr Rangan Chatterjee*, 8 March. Available at: https://open.spotify.com/episode/0uPpMRWwyDwUQfVyYrL1p8?si=9063a4e0ea9c4b9e
33. Ronald, I. (2022). 'Olympic medalist Dina Asher-Smith calls for more research into how periods affect athletic performance', *CNN*, 19 August. Available at: https://edition.cnn.com/2022/08/19/sport/dina-asher-smith-periods-performance-research-spt-intl/index.html
34. BBC Sport (2022). *Female athletes back #SayPeriod campaign*, 25 October. Available at: https://www.bbc.co.uk/sport/63371321
35. Guardian sport (2022). *Wimbledon will allow dark undershorts due to female players' period concerns*, 17 November. Available at: https://www.theguardian.com/sport/2022/nov/17/wimbledon-allow-dark-undershorts-due-to-female-players-period-concerns-tennis
36. Frye, A. (2024). 'Megan Rapinoe encourages women: sport your period', *Forbes*, 18 July. Available at: https://www.forbes.com/sites/andyfrye/2024/07/18/megan-rapinoe-encourages-women-sport-your-period/

37. Ronca, F., Watson, E., Metcalf, I. et al. (2025). 'Menstrual cycle and athletic status interact to influence symptoms, mood, and cognition in females', *Sports Medicine - Open*, 11, 104. doi: 10.1186/s40798-025-00924-8.
38. Gupta, A. H. (2023). 'Can cycle syncing benefit your workout? What experts say', *The New York Times*, 1 June. Available at: https://www.nytimes.com/2023/06/01/well/move/menstrual-cycle-syncing-exercise.html
39. Pasha-Robinson, L. (2017). 'Nearly half of girls do not know what is happening when they start their first period, study reveals', *The Independent*, 21 March. Available at: https://www.independent.co.uk/life-style/health-and-families/health-news/girls-teenagers-start-period-menstruation-education-women-s-health-betty-for-schools-a7636246.html
40. World Health Organization (2025). *Endometriosis*, 15 October. Available at: https://www.who.int/news-room/fact-sheets/detail/endometriosis
41. Endometriosis UK (no date). *Endometriosis facts and figures*. Available at: https://www.endometriosis-uk.org/endometriosis-facts-and-figures
42. Hunt, E. (2017). '"Enjoy menstruation, even on the subway": Stockholm art sparks row', *The Guardian*, 2 November. Available at: https://www.theguardian.com/cities/2017/nov/02/enjoy-menstruation-subway-stockholm-art-row-liv-stromquist
43. Martinčič, J. (2016). 'Let it bleed – art's revival of menstrual blood', *The Guardian*, 12 December. Available at: https://www.theguardian.com/lifeandstyle/2016/dec/12/let-it-bleed-arts-revival-of-menstrual-blood

44. Carrara, V. (2022). 'Easy menstrual blood plant fertilizer for Plastic Free July', *Ruby Cup*, 7 July. Available at: https://rubycup.com/blogs/news/easy-menstrual-blood-plant-fertilizer-for-plastic-free-july
45. DeFino, J. (2020). 'I tried a period-blood face mask and, uh, you definitely shouldn't', *Cosmopolitan*, 6 February. Available at: https://www.cosmopolitan.com/style-beauty/beauty/a30778631/menstrual-masking-period-blood-face-mask/
46. Hivemind, M. (2017). 'Menstrual Blood Magic - 13 Ways to Use Your Period in Spells', *Mookychick*, 5 August. Available at: https://www.mookychick.co.uk/health/witchcraft-spirituality/blood-magic-ways-to-use-menstrual-blood-in-magic-spells-and-ritual.php
47. Trueheart, L. (2019). 'Abso-bloody-lutely: Five uses for your period blood every month', *Dazed*, 12 November. Available at: https://www.dazeddigital.com/beauty/article/46784/1/uses-for-period-blood-beauty-face-mask-nail-polish-menstrual-cycle
48. Stardust, L. (2019). 'Menstrual Blood Magic: 3 Spells for your Period', *Teen Vogue*, 17 September. Available at: https://www.teenvogue.com/story/menstrual-blood-magic

Chapter 3

1. Collins, N. (2018). 'Demi's big moment', Vanity Fair, 16 April. Available at: https://www.vanityfair.com/style/2018/04/demi-moore-cover-story-august-1991

2. Duff, A. (2018). 'The Queen "thinks the word pregnant is vulgar" and prefers to say women are "in the family way", reveals royal insider', *The Sun*, 26 November. Available at: https://www.thesun.co.uk/fabulous/7832143/the-queen-word-pregnant-vulgar-different-term/
3. Gadsden, S. (2022). 'Coercion and reasons not to home birth', *Caerphilly Doula*, 22 November. Available at: https://caerphillydoula.co.uk/homebirth/coercion-reasons-not-to-home-birth/
4. NICE (no date). *Planning place of birth*. Available at: https://www.nice.org.uk/guidance/ng235/chapter/Recommendations#planning-place-of-birth
5. Atwood, M. (2024). *The Handmaid's Tale*. London: Vintage.
6. Olivia Downs (no date). Available at: https://www.tiktok.com/@lvdwns/video/7138442699786505518?lang=en
7. Sherman, C. (2025). 'Permanent contraception and abortion: Roe v Wade', *The Guardian*, 6 January. Available at: https://www.theguardian.com/us-news/2025/jan/06/permanent-contraception-abortion-roe-v-wade
8. TikTok (no date). 'TikTok video' [video]. Available at: https://www.tiktok.com/t/ZP8FWD5ne/
9. World Bank Open Data. (no date). *World Bank Open Data*. [online] Available at: https://data.worldbank.org/indicator/SP.DYN.TFRT.IN?.
10. Gonsalves, E. (2023) 30 November. Available at: https://www.instagram.com/p/C0Q2icHuEck/
11. McLaughlin, C. (2023). 'I shared a list of 117 reasons I don't want children. The response reiterated my point', *Mamamia*,

27 November. Available at: https://www.mamamia.com.au/ellie-gonsalves-child-free-list

12. BBC News (2021). *Poland clarifies abortion law after protests over mother's death*, 8 November. Available at: https://www.bbc.co.uk/news/world-europe-59206683
13. Tilles, D. (2022). 'Woman dies in Poland after having to carry dead foetus for seven days', *Notes from Poland*, 26 January. Available at: https://notesfrompoland.com/2022/01/26/woman-dies-in-poland-after-being-made-to-carry-dead-foetus-for-seven-days/
14. Wikipedia (no date). *Death of Amber Thurman*. Available at: https://en.wikipedia.org/wiki/Death_of_Amber_Thurman
15. Turner, B. and Hill, M. (2014). '"Kidnapped" by the authorities: meet the woman forced to have a caesarean', *The Telegraph*, 17 April. Available at: https://www.telegraph.co.uk/women/mother-tongue/10767161/Kidnapped-by-the-authorities-meet-the-woman-forced-to-have-a-caesarean.html
16. Carlisle, M. (2022). 'Fetal personhood laws are a new frontier in the battle over reproductive rights', *TIME*, 28 June. Available at: https://time.com/6191886/fetal-personhood-laws-roe-abortion/
17. Martin, E. (1991). 'The Egg and the Sperm: How Science Has Constructed a Romance Based on Stereotypical Male-Female Roles', *Signs: Journal of Women in Culture and Society*, 16(3), pp.485–501. doi: 10.1086/494680.
18. Druet, A. (2017). 'What is ovulation? Signs, symptoms and science', *Clue*, 30 November. Available at: https://helloclue.com/articles/cycle-a-z/ovulation-101-what-is-it-how-does-it-work

19. Cleveland Clinic (2022). 'Fimbriae', *Cleveland Clinic*, 25 October. Available at: https://my.clevelandclinic.org/health/body/24346-fimbriae#
20. Jabr, F. (2011). 'How human eggs woo sperm', *New Scientist*, 16 March. Available at: https://www.newscientist.com/article/mg20928043-400-how-human-eggs-woo-sperm/
21. Give Legacy (2022). *Does the sperm choose the egg — or does the egg choose the sperm?*, 5 May. Available at: https://www.givelegacy.com/resources/does-the-sperm-choose-the-egg-or-does-the-egg-choose-the-sperm/
22. University of Manchester (2020). *Human eggs prefer some men's sperm over others, research shows*, 10 June. Available at: https://www.manchester.ac.uk/discover/news/human-eggs-prefer-some-mens-sperm-over-others-research-shows/
23. Dalton, L. (2022). 'Understanding the female reproductive tract's role in fertilization', *ACS Central Science*, 8(1), pp. 3–6. doi: 10.1021/acscentsci.1c01595.
24. Repschläger, C. (2020). 'Female's cervical mucus selects best sperm', *Progress*, 24 August. Available at: https://www.progress.org.uk/females-cervical-mucus-selects-best-sperm/
25. Alberts, B., Johnson, A., Lewis, J., Raff, M., Roberts, K. and Walter, P. (2002). 'Fertilization', *Molecular Biology of the Cell*. Available at: https://www.ncbi.nlm.nih.gov/books/NBK26843/#
26. Gilbert, S. F. and Correia, C. P. (2017). *Fear, Wonder, and Science in the New Age of Reproductive Biotechnology*. New York: Columbia University Press.
27. Cheeseman, L. P., Boulanger, J., Bond, L. M. and Schuh, M. (2016). 'Two pathways regulate cortical granule translocation

to prevent polyspermy in mouse oocytes', *Nature Communications*, 7(1). doi: 10.1038/ncomms13726.

28. Condon, O. (2018). 'The diagram that shows how little women speak in Oscar-winning movies', *Her*, 6 March. Available at: https://www.her.ie/entertainment/diagram-shows-little-women-speak-oscar-winning-movies-392555
29. Williams, M. (2012). '"Legitimate rape" rarely leads to pregnancy, claims US Senate candidate', *The Guardian*, 19 August. Available at: https://www.theguardian.com/world/2012/aug/19/republican-todd-akin-rape-pregnancy
30. Heggie, V. (2012). '"Legitimate rape" – a medieval medical concept', *The Guardian*, 20 August. Available at: https://www.theguardian.com/science/the-h-word/2012/aug/20/legitimate-rape-medieval-medical-concept
31. Wilson, C. (1998). 'Seeing Things', *London Review of Books*, 12 May. Available at: https://www.lrb.co.uk/the-paper/v20/n10/catherine-wilson/seeing-things
32. NHS (2022). *Is it safe to use a sauna or jacuzzi if I'm pregnant?*, 26 July. Available at: https://www.nhs.uk/common-health-questions/pregnancy/is-it-safe-to-use-a-sauna-or-jacuzzi-if-i-am-pregnant/
33. Vihavainen, R. (no date). 'Sauna and health effects', *The Finnish Sauna Society*. Available at: https://sauna.fi/en/sauna-knowledge/sauna-and-health-effects/
34. The National Archives (2007). *Updated alcohol advice for pregnant women*, 26 May. Available at: https://webarchive.nationalarchives.gov.uk/ukgwa/+/www.direct.gov.uk/en/Nl1/Newsroom/DG_068143

35. National Childbirth Trust (2021). *Alcohol: Can I drink when I'm pregnant?*, 17 March. Available at: https://www.nct.org.uk/pregnancy/food-and-nutrition/alcohol-can-i-drink-when-im-pregnant
36. Illig, K. F. (2016). 'Barista refuses to serve coffee to a pregnant woman', *Redbook*, 29 January. Available at: https://www.redbookmag.com/body/pregnancy-fertility/a42239/come-again-now/
37. Rush, J. (2013). '"I refuse to have serving alcohol to pregnant women on my conscience": What bartender "told humiliated banker after she asked for a small glass of red wine"', *Daily Mail*, 27 September. Available at: https://www.dailymail.co.uk/news/article-2434739/I-refuse-serving-alcohol-pregnant-women-conscience--What-bartender-told-humiliated-mother-asked-small-glass-red-wine.html
38. Old Square Chambers (2014). *Foetal alcohol damages case dismissed by Court of Appeal*, 4 December. Available at: https://oldsquare.co.uk/foetal-alcohol-damages-case-dismissed-by-court-of-appeal/
39. Swindells, K. (2021). 'Why are so many pregnant women in hospital with Covid19', *New Statesman*, September. Available at: https://www.newstatesman.com/science-tech/2021/09/why-are-so-many-pregnant-women-in-hospital-with-covid-19
40. Royal, T. (2012). 'Whenua – the placenta', *Te Ara*, 22 September. Available at: https://teara.govt.nz/en/papatuanuku-the-land/page-4

41. Pohlmann, B. (2022). *Honoring the Placenta (Ari-Ari) Ritual in Bali and Indonesia* [online video], 21 November. Available at: https://www.youtube.com/watch?v=5_RyG7JPCU8
42. de Bellefonds, C. (no date). 'What is the placenta — and how does it help your baby grow?', *What to Expect*. Available at: https://www.whattoexpect.com/pregnancy/placenta (last updated 9 Oct 2025)
43. Martone, R. (2012). 'Scientists discover children's cells living in mothers' brains', *Scientific American*, 4 December. Available at: https://www.scientificamerican.com/article/scientists-discover-childrens-cells-living-in-mothers-brain/
44. Chan, W. F. N., Gurnot, C., Montine, T. J., Sonnen, J. A., Guthrie, K. A. and Nelson, J. L. (2012). 'Male microchimerism in the human female brain', *PLoS ONE*, 7(9), e45592. doi: 10.1371/journal.pone.0045592.
45. Zhou, L., Yoshimura, Y., Huang, Y., Suzuki, R., Yokoyama, M., Okabe, M. and Shimamura, M. (2000). 'Two independent pathways of maternal cell transmission to offspring: through placenta during pregnancy and by breast-feeding after birth', *Immunology*, 101(4), pp. 570–580. doi: 10.1046/j.1365-2567.2000.00144.x.
46. Bakar, F. (2023). 'Myleene Klass shares poignant message about miscarriages', *Metro*, 6 March. Available at: https://metro.co.uk/2023/03/06/myleene-klass-shares-poignant-message-about-miscarriages-18382616/
47. Yong, E. (2015). 'Foetal cells hide out in mum's body, but what do they do?', *National Geographic*, 7 September. Available at: https://www.nationalgeographic.com/science/

article/foetal-cells-hide-out-in-mums-body-but-what-do-they-do

48. Tucker, A. (2021). 'Moms: You shaped your children, but the reverse is true, too — down to your very cells', *Washington Post*, 6 May. Available at: https://www.washingtonpost.com/lifestyle/2021/05/06/motherhood-biology-fetus-change-microchimerism/
49. Kara, R. J., Bolli, P., Karakikes, I., Matsunaga, I., Tripodi, J., Tanweer, O., Altman, P., Shachter, N. S., Nakano, A., Najfeld, V. and Chaudhry, H. W. (2011). 'Fetal cells traffic to injured maternal myocardium and undergo cardiac differentiation', *Circulation Research*, 110(1), pp. 82–93. doi: 10.1161/circresaha.111.249037.
50. McCormack, C., Callaghan, B. L. and Pawluski, J. L. (2023). 'It's time to rebrand "Mommy Brain"', *JAMA Neurology*, 80(4), p. 335. doi: 10.1001/jamaneurol.2022.5180.
51. Hoekzema, E., Tamnes, C. K., Berns, P., Barba-Müller, E., Pozzobon, C., Picado, M., Lucco, F., Martínez-García, M., Desco, M., Ballesteros, A., Crone, E. A., Vilarroya, O. and Carmona, S. (2020). 'Becoming a mother entails anatomical changes in the ventral striatum of the human brain that facilitate its responsiveness to offspring cues', *Psychoneuroendocrinology*, 112, 104507. doi: 10.1016/j.psyneuen.2019.104507.
52. Callaghan, B., McCormack, C., Tottenham, N. and Monk, C. (2022). 'Evidence for cognitive plasticity during pregnancy via enhanced learning and memory', Memory, 30(5), pp. 519–536. doi: 10.1080/09658211.2021.2019280.

53. Carmona, S., Martínez-García, M., Paternina-Die, M., Barba-Müller, E., Wierenga, L. M., Alemán-Gómez, Y., Pretus, C., Marcos-Vidal, L., Beumala, L., Cortizo, R., Pozzobon, C., Picado, M., Lucco, F., García-García, D., Soliva, J. C., Tobeña, A., Peper, J. S., Crone, E. A., Ballesteros, A., Vilarroya, O., Desco, M. and Hoekzema, E. (2019). 'Pregnancy and adolescence entail similar neuroanatomical adaptations: A comparative analysis of cerebral morphometric changes', *Human Brain Mapping*, 40(7), pp. 2143–2152. doi: 10.1002/hbm.24513.

Chapter 4

1. Kitzinger, S. (1978). *Women as Mothers*. Oxford: M. Robertson.
2. Beck, C. T., Watson, S. and Gable, R. K. (2018). 'Traumatic childbirth and its aftermath: Is there anything positive?', *The Journal of Perinatal Education*, 27(3), pp. 175–184. doi: 10.1891/1058-1243.27.3.175.
3. The Farm Midwifery Center (no date). *Preliminary statistics*. Available at: https://thefarmmidwives.org/preliminary-statistics/
4. March of Dimes (no date). *Total Cesarean deliveries by maternal race: United States, 2020–2022 average*. Available at: https://www.marchofdimes.org/peristats/data?reg=99&top=8&stop=355&lev=1&slev=1&obj=1
5. Clegg, R. (2025). 'Caesarean sections overtake natural vaginal births for the first time', *BBC News*, 17 December.

Available at: https://www.bbc.co.uk/news/articles/c5yqjezrnj4o

6. Davis, J. (2014). *Albany Midwifery Practice*. Available at: https://www.aims.org.uk/journal/item/albany-midwifery-practice
7. Reed, B. and Edwards, N. (no date). 'The rise and fall of the Albany Midwifery Practice, London 1997–2009', *Maternity and Midwifery*. Available at: https://maternityandmidwifery.co.uk/the-rise-and-fall-of-the-albany-midwifery-practice-london-1997-2009/
8. Press Association (2013). 'Panda pregnancy: Edinburgh Zoo put on 24-hour alert for Tian Tian', *The Guardian*, 26 August. Available at: https://www.theguardian.com/world/2013/aug/26/panda-pregnancy-edinburgh-tian-alert
9. Zhang, J., Landy, H. J., Branch, D. W., Burkman, R., Haberman, S., Gregory, K. D., Hatjis, C. G., Ramirez, M. M., Bailit, J. L., Gonzalez-Quintero, V. H., Hibbard, J. U., Hoffman, M. K., Kominiarek, M., Learman, L. A., Van Veldhuisen, P., Troendle, J. and Reddy, U. M. (2010). 'Contemporary patterns of spontaneous labor with normal neonatal outcomes', *Obstetrics and Gynecology*, 116(6), pp. 1281–1287. doi: 10.1097/AOG.0b013e3181fdef6e.
10. Reed, R. (2015). 'Vaginal examinations: stuck on the cervix', *Rachel Reed*, 2 May. Available at: https://www.rachelreed.website/blog/vaginal-examinations-in-labour
11. Moncrieff, G., Gyte, G. M., Dahlen, H. G., Thomson, G., Singata-Madliki, M., Clegg, A. and Downe, S. (2022). 'Routine vaginal examinations compared to other methods for assessing progress of labour to improve outcomes

for women and babies at term', *Cochrane Database of Systematic Reviews*, 2022(3). doi: 10.1002/14651858.CD010088.pub3.

12. Shepherd, A., Cheyne, H., Kennedy, S., McIntosh, C., Styles, M. and Niven, C. (2010). 'The purple line as a measure of labour progress: a longitudinal study', *BMC Pregnancy and Childbirth*, 10(1). doi: 10.1186/1471-2393-10-54.
13. Wickham, S. (2023). 'The Rhombus of Michaelis', Dr Sara Wickham, 16 March. Available at: https://www.sarawickham.com/articles-2/the-rhombus-of-michaelis/
14. Prins, M., Boxem, J., Lucas, C. and Hutton, E. (2011). 'Effect of spontaneous pushing versus Valsalva pushing in the second stage of labour on mother and fetus: a systematic review of randomised trials', *BJOG*, 118(6), pp. 662–670. doi: 10.1111/j.1471-0528.2011.02910.x.
15. Encyclopedia.com (no date). *Kristeller, Samuel*. Available at: https://www.encyclopedia.com/religion/encyclopedias-almanacs-transcripts-and-maps/kristeller-samuel
16. Thompson, A. (2019). 'Outdated, dangerous childbirth methods remain common in Europe', *Voice of America*, 26 December. Available at: https://learningenglish.voanews.com/a/outdated-dangerous-childbirth-methods-remain-common-in-europe/5204422.html
17. Gil, J., Rodríguez, J. M., Hernández, Q., González, M. and Torregrosa, N. (2021). 'Hemoperitoneum and the Kristeller maneuver', *Cirugía Española*, 99(6), pp. 468–469. doi: 10.1016/j.cireng.2020.06.014.
18. Willyard, C. (2020). 'Episiotomy rates are dropping, but some doctors still snip', *The New York Times*, 17 April.

Available at: https://www.nytimes.com/2020/04/17/parenting/episiotomy.html

19. Goueslard, K., Cottenet, J., Roussot, A., Clesse, C., Sagot, P. and Quantin, C. (2018). 'How did episiotomy rates change from 2007 to 2014? Population-based study in France', *BMC Pregnancy and Childbirth*, 18(1). doi: 10.1186/s12884-018-1747-8.
20. Yang, J. and Bai, H. (2021). 'Knowledge, attitude and experience of episiotomy practice among obstetricians and midwives: a cross-sectional study from China', *BMJ Open*, 11(4), e043596. doi: 10.1136/bmjopen-2020-043596.
21. Christophe, C., Jonathan, C., Joelle, L., Karine, G., Michele, S., Paul, S. and Catherine, Q. (2020). 'Episiotomy practices in France: epidemiology and risk factors in non-operative vaginal deliveries', Scientific Reports, 10(1). doi: 10.1038/s41598-020-70881-7.
22. Jiang, H., Qian, X., Carroli, G. and Garner, P. (2017). 'Selective versus routine use of episiotomy for vaginal birth', *Cochrane Database of Systematic Reviews*, 2017(2). doi: 10.1002/14651858.CD000081.pub3.
23. Ami, O., Maran, J. C., Gabor, P., Whitacre, E. B., Musset, D., Dubray, C., Mage, G. and Boyer, L. (2019). 'Three-dimensional magnetic resonance imaging of fetal head molding and brain shape changes during the second stage of labor', *PLOS ONE*, 14(5), e0215721. doi: 10.1371/journal.pone.0215721.
24. Richardson, H. (2019). 'Doctor claims that obese women with "fatter vaginas" are more likely to experience obstructed births', *Daily Mail*, 13 November. Available at:

https://www.dailymail.co.uk/femail/article-7680527/Doctor-claims-obese-women-fatter-vaginas-likely-experience-obstructed-births.html

25. Dunsworth, H. (2021). 'There is no evolutionary "obstetrical dilemma"', in Tomori, C. and Han, S. (eds.) *The Routledge Handbook of Anthropology and Reproduction*. Taylor & Francis. Available at: https://digitalcommons.uri.edu/cgi/viewcontent.cgi?article=1040&context=soc_facpubs
26. Odent, M. (1987). 'The Fetus Ejection Reflex', Birth, 14(2), pp. 104–105. doi: 10.1111/j.1523-536x.1987.tb01463.x.
27. Odent, M. (2015). *Do we need midwives?*. London: Pinter & Martin Ltd.
28. Awford, J. (2019). 'Top docs doubt "geriatric parent" Meghan will be able to have natural "doula and willow tree" birth', *The Sun*, 6 May. Available at: https://www.thesun.co.uk/fabulous/9010498/meghan-markle-home-birth-plan-is-mocked-top-docs/
29. Holland, K. (2018). 'Are middle-class "birthzillas" harassing hospital staff?', *The Irish Times*, 4 May. Available at: https://www.irishtimes.com/news/social-affairs/are-middle-class-birthzillas-harassing-hospital-staff-1.3484471
30. Lee, C. (2023). 5 September. Available at: https://x.com/ClementLeeMD/status/1699071108891410593
31. Thornton, J. (2019). 'Waterbirth videos', *Ripe-Tomato.org*, 7 February. Available at: https://ripe-tomato.org/2019/02/07/waterbirth-videos/
32. Skeptical OB (2017). *Milli Hill, 'queen of childbirth' gaslighting*. Available at: https://www.skepticalob.com/2017/03/milli-hill-queen-of-childbirth-gaslighting.html

33. The Mule (no date). *Arrogant doctors and rug doctors.* Available at: https://themule.substack.com/p/arrogant-doctors-and-rug-doctors
34. Mikkelson, D. (2019). 'Did Pat Robertson say feminism encourages women to "kill their children"?', *Snopes*, 4 April. Available at: https://www.snopes.com/fact-check/pat-robertson-feminist-agenda/
35. Mobbs, N., Williams, C. and Weeks, A. (2018). 'Humanising birth: Does the language we use matter?', *BMJ Opinion*, 8 February. Available at: https://blogs.bmj.com/bmj/2018/02/08/humanising-birth-does-the-language-we-use-matter/
36. Bowes, C. (2012). 'Janet Balaskas: campaigner for active birth movement', *BBC News*, 4 April. Available at: https://www.bbc.co.uk/news/health-17589544?app-referrer=deep-link
37. Mills, J. (2016). 'More than 1 in 20 women claim to orgasm while giving birth, survey shows', *Metro*, 11 December. Available at: https://metro.co.uk/2016/05/06/more-than-1-in-20-women-claim-to-orgasm-while-giving-birth-survey-shows-5864621/
38. Jowitt, M. (2018). 'Electronic fetal monitoring is more important than freedom of maternal position in labour', *BJOG*, 125(7), p. 894. doi: 10.1111/1471-0528.15026.
39. Wickham, S. (2023). 'The Rhombus of Michaelis', *Dr Sara Wickham*, 16 March. Available at: https://www.sarawickham.com/articles-2/the-rhombus-of-michaelis/
40. Kitzinger, S. (2012). Birth & Sex: The Power and the Passion. London: Pinter & Martin Ltd.

41. Pirdel, M. and Pirdel, L. (2009). 'Perceived environmental stressors and pain perception during labor among primiparous and multiparous women', *Journal of Reproduction & Infertility*, 1 December. Available at: https://www.ncbi.nlm.nih.gov/pmc/articles/PMC3719331/
42. Whitburn, L. Y., Jones, L. E., Davey, M. A. and Small, R. (2017). 'The meaning of labour pain: how the social environment and other contextual factors shape women's experiences', *BMC Pregnancy and Childbirth*, 17(1). doi: 10.1186/s12884-017-1343-3.
43. Van Der Gucht, N., Lewis, K. and University of Huddersfield Repository (2015). 'Women's experiences of coping with pain during childbirth: A critical review of qualitative research', *Midwifery*, 31, pp. 349–358. Available at: https://eprints.hud.ac.uk/id/eprint/23158/1/submitted_paper_adjusted.pdf

Chapter 5

1. Collins, L. (2022). 'The hidden mothers of family photos', *The New Yorker*, 12 February. Available at: https://www.newyorker.com/culture/culture-desk/the-hidden-mothers-of-family-photos
2. Dictionary.com (2023). *Why do babies around the world say "Mama"?*, 11 May. Available at: https://www.dictionary.com/e/mama/
3. Erard, M. (2019). 'How do people communicate before death?', *The Atlantic*, 16 January. Available at: https://www.theatlantic.com/family/archive/2019/01/how-do-people-communicate-before-death/580303/

4. BBC News (2020). *Freddy McConnell: Transgender man's bid to be named father fails*, 29 April. Available at: https://www.bbc.co.uk/news/uk-england-kent-52471697
5. Green, J. (2023). 'Emotional moment parents meet their surrogate baby boy in war-torn Ukraine as documentary exposes how the black market of commercial surrogacy is thriving', *Daily Mail*, 24 March. Available at: https://www.dailymail.co.uk/femail/real-life/article-11898411/Watch-moment-parents-meet-baby-boy-surrogate-war-torn-Ukraine.html
6. Kramer, A. E. (2020). '100 babies stranded in Ukraine after surrogate births', *The New York Times*, 18 September. Available at: https://www.nytimes.com/2020/05/16/world/europe/ukraine-coronavirus-surrogate-babies.html
7. Research and Markets (2025). 'Surrogacy Market Growth Drivers, Industry Trend Analysis and Forecast 2025–2034: Rapid Growth Expected in Below35 Segment Driven by Higher IVF Success Rates', *GlobeNewswire*, 23 April. Available at: https://www.globenewswire.com/news-release/2025/04/23/3066143/0/en/Surrogacy-Market-Growth-Drivers-Industry-Trend-Analysis-and-Forecast-2025-2034-Rapid-Growth-Expected-in-Below-35-Segment-Driven-by-Higher-IVF-Success-Rates.html
8. Gill, M. (2026). 'It's tragic that some women can't conceive – but surrogacy is too risky an answer', *The Observer*, 28 January. Available at: https://observer.co.uk/news/opinion-and-ideas/article/its-tragic-that-some-women-cant-conceive-but-surrogacy-is-too-risky-an-answer

9. Surrogacy Concern (2025). *Surrogacy Concern warmly welcomes presentation of UNSRVAWs report at the UN General Assembly calling for an international surrogacy ban*, 10 October. Available at: https://surrogacyconcern.uk/2025/10/10/surrogacy-concern-warmly-welcomes-presentation-of-unsrvaws-report-at-the-un-general-assembly-calling-for-an-international-surrogacy-ban/
10. Kendal, E. and Bhatia, N. (2019). 'We may one day grow babies outside the womb, but there are many things to consider first', *The Conversation*, 10 November. Available at: https://theconversation.com/we-may-one-day-grow-babies-outside-the-womb-but-there-are-many-things-to-consider-first-125709
11. Smajdor, A. (2022). 'Whole body gestational donation', *Theoretical Medicine and Bioethics*, 44(2), pp. 113–124. doi: 10.1007/s11017-022-09599-8.
12. NICE (2015). *Quality Statement 6: Delayed cord clamping*, 10 December. Available at: https://www.nice.org.uk/guidance/qs105/chapter/Quality-statement-6-Delayed-cord-clamping
13. Andersson, O. and Zaigham, M. (2023). 'Cord clamping – "hold on a minute" is not enough, and sample your blood gases while waiting', *Seminars in Perinatology*, 47(4), 151739. doi: 10.1016/j.semperi.2023.151739.
14. Amanda (2020). 'Primal birth', *Wait for White*, 19 February. Available at: https://waitforwhite.com/primal-birth/
15. Hodousek, C. (2022). 'WV med student delivers wife's baby in car during Utah snow storm', WV *MetroNews*, 28 January. Available at: https://wvmetronews.com/2022/01/28/

wv-med-student-delivers-wifes-baby-in-car-during-utah-snow-storm/

16. Adopstar (2021). 'Officers reunited with baby they delivered in the street', *Jersey Evening Post*, 9 September. Available at: https://www.jerseyeveningpost.com/morenews/uknews/2021/09/09/officers-reunited-with-baby-they-delivered-in-the-street/
17. Andersson, O., Hellström-Westas, L., Andersson, D. and Domellöf, M. (2011). 'Effect of delayed versus early umbilical cord clamping on neonatal outcomes and iron status at 4 months: a randomised controlled trial', *British Medical Journal*, 343(nov15 1), d7157. doi: 10.1136/bmj.d7157.
18. Andersson, O., Lindquist, B., Lindgren, M., Stjernqvist, K., Domellöf, M. and Hellström-Westas, L. (2015). 'Effect of delayed cord clamping on neurodevelopment at 4 years of age', *JAMA Pediatrics*, 169(7), p. 631. doi: 10.1001/jamapediatrics.2015.0358.
19. Rabe, H., Gyte, G. M., DíazRossello, J. L. and Duley, L. (2019). 'Effect of timing of umbilical cord clamping and other strategies to influence placental transfusion at preterm birth on maternal and infant outcomes', *Cochrane Database of Systematic Reviews*, 2019(9). doi: 10.1002/14651858.CD003248.pub4.
20. Boere, I., Roest, A. a. W., Wallace, E., Harkel, A. D. J. T., Haak, M. C., Morley, C. J., Hooper, S. B. and Pas, A. B. T. (2014). 'Umbilical blood flow patterns directly after birth before delayed cord clamping', *Archives of Disease in Childhood. Fetal and Neonatal Edition*, 100(2), F121–F125. doi: 10.1136/archdischild-2014-307144.

21. Palethorpe, R. J., Farrar, D. and Duley, L. (2010). 'Alternative positions for the baby at birth before clamping the umbilical cord', *Cochrane Database of Systematic Reviews*, 2012(2). doi: 10.1002/14651858.CD007555.pub2.
22. WallerWise, R. (2011). 'Umbilical cord blood: Information for childbirth educators', The Journal of Perinatal Education, 20(1), pp. 54–60. doi: 10.1891/1058-1243.20.1.54.
23. Zhang, S. (2022). 'Don't pay for cordblood banking', *The Atlantic*, 17 October. Available at: https://www.theatlantic.com/health/archive/2022/10/cord-blood-banking-transplant-cost-worth-it/671765/
24. Widström, A., Brimdyr, K., Svensson, K., Cadwell, K. and Nissen, E. (2019). 'Skintoskin contact the first hour after birth, underlying implications and clinical practice', *Acta Paediatrica*, 108(7), pp. 1192–1204. doi: 10.1111/apa.14754.
25. Chiruvolu, A., Miklis, K. K., Stanzo, K. C., Petrey, B., Groves, C. G., McCord, K., Qin, H., Desai, S. and Tolia, V. N. (2017). 'Effects of skintoskin care on late preterm and term infants atrisk for neonatal hypoglycemia', *Pediatric Quality & Safety*, 2(4), e030. doi: 10.1097/pq9.0000000000000030.
26. UNICEF (2018). *Breastfeeding from the first hour of birth: What works and what hurts*, 31 July. Available at: https://www.unicef.org/stories/breastfeeding-first-hour-birth-what-works-and-what-hurts
27. Alderson, S. (2014). 'Skin to skin', *Fab NHS Stuff*, 25 December. Available at: https://fabnhsstuff.net/fab-stuff/story76

28. Infant Feeding Alliance (2023). *Skin to skin: the baby isn't the only one in their birthday suit*, 19 January. Available at: https://www.infantfeedingalliance.org.uk/2023/01/19/skin-to-skin-the-baby-isnt-the-only-one-in-their-birthday-suit/
29. Fed Is Best Foundation (no date). *Category: Baby-Friendly Protocol Complications: Starvation, Jaundice, Hypoglycemia, Dehydration, Newborn Falls.* Available at: https://fedisbest.org/category/baby-friendly-hospital-complications/
30. Williams, S. (2024). Available at: https://www.instagram.com/p/C3P_-9QO-4O/
31. Baldwin, I. (2026). 'Serena Williams weight loss – Super Bowl', *Daily Mail*, 29 January. Available at: https://www.dailymail.co.uk/sport/tennis/article-15507431/serena-williams-weight-loss-super-bowl.html
32. Hodgkinson, E. L., Smith, D. M. and Wittkowski, A. (2014). 'Women's experiences of their pregnancy and postpartum body image: a systematic review and metasynthesis', *BMC Pregnancy and Childbirth*, 14(1). doi: 10.1186/1471-2393-14-330.
33. Brown, A., Rance, J. and Warren, L. (2015). 'Body image concerns during pregnancy are associated with a shorter breastfeeding duration', *Midwifery*, 31(1), pp. 80–89. doi: 10.1016/j.midw.2014.06.003.
34. Thomas, K. (2022). 'New study reveals the public make it more difficult for women to breastfeed', Swansea University News, 2 August. Available at: https://www.swansea.ac.uk/press-office/news-events/news/2022/08/

new-study-reveals-the-public-make-it-more-difficult-for-women-to-breastfeed-.php

35. NHS (2023). *Breastfeeding in public*, 28 March. Available at: https://www.nhs.uk/conditions/baby/breastfeeding-and-bottle-feeding/breastfeeding/breastfeeding-in-public/#
36. Javed, S. (2022). 'Sainsbury's staffer told new mother it was "inappropriate" to breastfeed in car park', *The Independent*, 28 June. Available at: https://www.independent.co.uk/life-style/women/sainsburys-mother-breastfeed-public-baby-b2111190.html
37. Hinde, N. (2022). 'What's your problem with mums breastfeeding in public?', *HuffPost UK*, 25 October. Available at: https://www.huffingtonpost.co.uk/entry/stop-shaming-mums-for-breastfeeding-in-public_uk_6357a312e4b08e0e609230ae
38. Brazell, E. (2023). 'South Tyneside: Mum breastfeeding in swimming pool told "go near drain"', *Metro*, 26 March. Available at: https://metro.co.uk/2023/03/26/south-tyneside-mum-breastfeeding-in-swimming-pool-told-go-near-drain-18503972/
39. Warner, M. (2022). 'Should mums be allowed to breastfeed in swimming pools?', *Rhyl Journal*, 5 July. Available at: https://www.rhyljournal.co.uk/news/20254585.mums-allowed-breastfeed-swimming-pools/
40. Ballard, O. and Morrow, A. L. (2013). 'Human milk composition', *Pediatric Clinics of North America*, 60(1), pp. 49–74. doi: 10.1016/j.pcl.2012.10.002.

41. Underwood, M. A. (2013). 'Human milk for the premature infant', *Pediatric Clinics of North America*, 60(1), pp. 189–207. doi: 10.1016/j.pcl.2012.09.008.
42. CzosnykowskaŁukacka, M., LisKuberka, J., KrólakOlejnik, B. and OrczykPawiłowicz, M. (2020). 'Changes in human milk immunoglobulin profile during prolonged lactation', *Frontiers in Pediatrics*, 8. doi: 10.3389/fped.2020.00428.
43. Geddes, L. (2009). 'Evening breast milk means a good sleep', *New Scientist*, 2 October. Available at: https://www.newscientist.com/article/dn17908-evening-breast-milk-means-a-good-sleep/
44. Butterfield, R. (2021). 'Breastfeeding at night', *La Leche League GB*, February. Available at: https://www.laleche.org.uk/breastfeeding-at-night/#
45. Newmark, L. (2022). 'Baby backwash can trigger immune response in milk', *International Milk Genomics Consortium*. Available at: https://www.milkgenomics.org/?splash=baby-backwash-can-trigger-immune-response-in-milk#
46. AlShehri, S. S., Knox, C. L., Liley, H. G., Cowley, D. M., Wright, J. R., Henman, M. G., Hewavitharana, A. K., Charles, B. G., Shaw, P. N., Sweeney, E. L. and Duley, J. A. (2015). 'Breastmilk–saliva interactions boost innate immunity by regulating the oral microbiome in early infancy', *PLOS ONE*, 10(9), e0135047. doi: 10.1371/journal.pone.0135047.
47. Hess, M. K., Hess, A. S. and Garrick, D. J. (2016). 'The effect of calf gender on milk production in seasonal calving cows and its impact on genetic evaluations', *PLOS ONE*, 11(3), e0151236. doi: 10.1371/journal.pone.0151236.

48. Koskela, E., Mappes, T., Niskanen, T. and Rutkowska, J. (2009). 'Maternal investment in relation to sex ratio and offspring number in a small mammal – a case for Trivers and Willard theory?', *Journal of Animal Ecology*, 78(5), pp. 1007–1014. doi: 10.1111/j.1365-2656.2009.01574.x.
49. Galante, L., Milan, A. M., Reynolds, C. M., CameronSmith, D., Vickers, M. H. and Pundir, S. (2018). 'Sexspecific human milk composition: The role of infant sex in determining early life nutrition', *Nutrients*, 10(9), 1194. doi: 10.3390/nu10091194.
50. Fox, R., McMullen, S. and Newburn, M. (2015). 'UK women's experiences of breastfeeding and additional breastfeeding support: a qualitative study of Baby Café services', *BMC Pregnancy and Childbirth*, 15(1). doi: 10.1186/s12884-015-0581-5.
51. Neifert, M. and Bunik, M. (2013). 'Overcoming clinical barriers to exclusive breastfeeding', *Pediatric Clinics of North America*, 60(1), pp. 115–145. doi: 10.1016/j.pcl.2012.10.001.
52. UNICEF UK (2022). 'Breastfeeding in the UK', 11 March. Available at: https://www.unicef.org.uk/babyfriendly/about/breastfeeding-in-the-uk/
53. CassarUhl, D. (2023). 'Perceived Insufficient Milk', *Kelly Mom*, 28 November. Available at: https://kellymom.com/bf/got-milk/perceived-insufficient-milk/
54. Nelson, A. (2018). 'The politics of breastfeeding (and why it must change)', *Forbes*, 24 October. Available at: https://www.forbes.com/sites/amynelson1/2018/10/24/the-politics-of-breastfeeding-and-why-it-must-change/

55. Rossin, M. (2011). 'The effects of maternity leave on children's birth and infant health outcomes in the United States', *Journal of Health Economics*, 30(2), pp. 221–239. doi: 10.1016/j.jhealeco.2011.01.005.
56. Campbell, D. (2022). 'Record numbers of women reach 30 childfree in England and Wales', *The Guardian*, 27 January. Available at: https://www.theguardian.com/lifeandstyle/2022/jan/27/women-child-free-30-ons
57. Brown, L. (2022). 'Regretting motherhood: What have I done to my life?', *Today's Parent*, 13 October. Available at: https://www.todaysparent.com/family/parenting/i-regret-motherhood/
58. Hughes, S. (2025). 'Unmasking the man behind toxic gossip website Tattle Life', *The Guardian*, 21 September. Available at: https://www.theguardian.com/society/2025/sep/21/unmasking-the-man-behind-toxic-gossip-website-tattle-life
59. Chiorando, M. and Hawken, L. (2023). 'Mummy blogger Clemmie Hooper receives oneyear caution order following midwifery misconduct hearing', *Daily Mail*, 7 March. Available at: https://www.dailymail.co.uk/femail/article-11831001/Mummy-blogger-Clemmie-Hooper-receives-one-year-caution-order-following-midwifery-misconduct-hearing.html
60. Dashú, M. (2020). 'Not Venus Figurines', *Suppressed Histories*. Available at: https://www.suppressedhistories.net/articles/notvenusfigurines.html
61. Acadamy HAGIA (no date). *Matriarchy*. Available at: https://hagia.de/en/matriarchy/

Chapter 6

1. NHS (2022). *Symptoms*, 17 May. Available at: https://www.nhs.uk/conditions/menopause/symptoms/
2. Landau, M. (2022). 'The Wild History of Women's Hormone Therapy', *Everyday Health*, 13 December. Available at: https://www.everydayhealth.com/womens-health/hormones/history-hormone-therapy/
3. Boswell, K. (no date). 'Heartbreaking truth about the treatment of horses used to produce estrogen replacement drugs', *One Green Planet*. Available at: https://www.onegreenplanet.org/animalsandnature/heartbreaking-truth-about-the-treatment-of-horses-used-to-produce-estrogen-replacement-drugs/
4. Wikipedia (2025). *Conjugated estrogens*. Available at: https://en.wikipedia.org/wiki/Conjugated_estrogens
5. Cagnacci, A. and Venier, M. (2019). 'The controversial history of hormone replacement therapy', *Medicina*, 55(9), p. 602. doi: 10.3390/medicina55090602.
6. Robinson, L. and BMS Medical Advisory Council (2020). 'HRT: The History', *Women's Health Concern*, November. Available at: https://www.womens-health-concern.org/wp-content/uploads/2022/11/10-WHC-FACTSHEET-HRT-The-history-NOV22-A.pdf
7. Royal Osteoporosis Society (2025). *Hormone replacement therapy (HRT)*. Available at: https://theros.org.uk/information-and-support/osteoporosis/treatment/hormone-replacement-therapy/
8. Taylor, J. E., Baig, M. S., Helmy, T. and Gersh, F. L. (2021). 'Controversies regarding postmenopausal hormone

replacement therapy for primary cardiovascular disease prevention in women', *Cardiology in Review*, 29(6), pp. 296–304. doi: 10.1097/CRD.0000000000000353.

9. BBC News (2023). *HRT could cut Alzheimer's risk in some women - early study*, 14 January. Available at: https://www.bbc.co.uk/news/health-64276452
10. Espeland, M. A., Hogan, P. E., Fineberg, S. E., Howard, G., Schrott, H., Waclawiw, M. A. and Bush, T. L. (1998). 'Effect of postmenopausal hormone therapy on glucose and insulin concentrations', *Diabetes Care*, 21(10), pp. 1589–1595. doi: 10.2337/diacare.21.10.1589.
11. Sator, P., Schmidt, J., Sator, M., Huber, J. and Hönigsmann, H. (2001). 'The influence of hormone replacement therapy on skin ageing', *Maturitas*, 39(1), pp. 43–55. doi: 10.1016/S0378-5122(00)00225-5.
12. NICE (2024). *Menopause: diagnosis and management*, 7 November. Available at: https://www.nice.org.uk/guidance/ng23/chapter/Recommendations#long-term-benefits-and-risks-of-hormone-replacement-therapy
13. Howard, S. (2021). 'Experimental treatments risk further medicalisation of menopause', *BMJ*, 373:n992. doi: 10.1136/bmj.n992.
14. SkyQuest (2024). *Hormone Replacement Therapy (HRT)*. Available at: https://www.skyquestt.com/report/hormone-replacement-therapy-market
15. Collings, J. (2021). 'The Connection between Menarche And Childbirth', *Jane Hardwicke Collings*, 6 February. Available at: https://janehardwickecollings.com/the-connection-between-menarche-and-childbirth/

16. Collings, J. (2021). 'Introducing Mage', *Jane Hardwicke Collings*, 6 February. Available at: https://janehardwickecollings.com/introducing-maga/
17. Warren, H. and Dubin, A. (1933) 'Keep Young and Beautiful'. [Recorded by Eddie Cantor]. *Roman Scandals Soundtrack*. [Vinyl]. Hollywood: Warner Bros.
18. MSN (no date). 'Pamela Anderson on redefining beauty on her own terms', MSN Lifestyle Buzz. Available at: https://www.msn.com/en-us/lifestyle/lifestyle-buzz/pamela-anderson-on-redefining-beauty-on-her-own-terms/
19. Bezzant, N. (2022). '"She will not become dull and unattractive": The charming history of menopause and HRT', *The Guardian*, 18 January. Available at: https://www.theguardian.com/world/2022/jan/18/she-will-not-become-dull-and-unattractive-the-charming-history-of-menopause-and-hrt
20. Moran, C. (2020). 'Caitlin Moran: me, drugs and the perimenopause', *The Times*, 3 July. Available at: https://www.thetimes.co.uk/article/caitlin-moran-me-drugs-and-the-perimenopause-mpzn2cdh2
21. Moore, S. (2015). 'There Won't Be Blood: Suzanne Moore on the menopause', *New Statesman*, 17 August. Available at: https://www.newstatesman.com/long-reads/2015/08/there-wont-be-blood-suzanne-moore-menopause
22. Wilson, R. (1966). *Feminine Forever*. [online] Open Library. Available at: https://openlibrary.org/works/OL7399848W/Feminine_Forever?edition=key%3A/books/OL5982073M
23. Dominus, S. (2023). 'Women have been misled about menopause', *The New York Times*, 15 June. Available at:

https://www.nytimes.com/2023/02/01/magazine/menopause-hot-flashes-hormone-therapy.html

24. Wikipedia (2025). *Robert Wilson*. Available at: https://en.wikipedia.org/wiki/Robert_A._Wilson_(gynecologist)
25. Adams, G. (2022). 'Glasgow Life defends trans label in Burrell Collection after "politicisation" row', *Museums Association*, 22 April. Available at: https://www.museumsassociation.org/museums-journal/news/2022/04/glasgow-life-defends-trans-label-in-the-burrell-collection-after-politicisation-row/#
26. Cherry, K. (2024). 'Joan of Arc: Cross-dressing warrior-saint and LGBTQ role model', *Q Spirit*, 5 May. Available at: https://qspirit.net/joan-of-arc-cross-dressing-lgbtq/ (last updated 1 Feb 2026)
27. DAY BY DAY Shoppe (2022) 27 June. Available at: https://www.facebook.com/mydaybydayshoppe/photos/a.885911851579857/2067530650084632/?type=3
28. NHS Business Services Authority (2022). *NHS publishes new HRT official statistics*, 6 October. Available at: https://media.nhsbsa.nhs.uk/news/nhs-publishes-new-hrt-official-statistics
29. Bryant, M. (2022). 'HRT demand expected to surge after new Davina McCall film on menopause', *The Guardian*, 1 May. Available at: https://www.theguardian.com/society/2022/may/01/hrt-demand-expected-to-surge-after-new-davina-mccall-film-on-menopause
30. Kollewe, J. (2022). 'HRT: inside the complex global supply chain behind a $20bn market', *The Guardian*, 24 September. Available at: https://www.theguardian.com/business/2022/sep/24/

hrt-inside-the-complex-global-supply-chain-behind-a-20bn-market

31. Centre for Ageing Better (no date). *Women in their 40s and 50s earning 20% less than their male peers, according to new figures*. Available at: https://ageing-better.org.uk/news/women-in-their-40s-and-50s-earning-less-than-their-male-peers
32. ITV News (2021). *Suicide rates in women of menopausal age rise*, 17 November. Available at: https://www.itv.com/news/2021-11-16/suicide-rates-in-women-of-menopausal-age-rise
33. Kulkarni, J. (2018). 'Perimenopausal depression – an under-recognised entity', *Australian Prescriber*, 41(6), pp. 183–185. doi: 10.18773/austprescr.2018.060.
34. UK Parliament Committees (2022). *Menopause and the workplace*, 28 July. Available at: https://committees.parliament.uk/work/1416/menopause-and-the-workplace/publications/
35. Bromberger, J. T. and Epperson, C. N. (2018). 'Depression during and after the perimenopause', *Obstetrics and Gynecology Clinics of North America*, 45(4), pp. 663–678. doi: 10.1016/j.ogc.2018.07.007.
36. Shea, A. K., Frey, B. N., Gervais, N., Lopez, A. and Minuzzi, L. (2021). 'Depression in midlife women attending a menopause clinic is associated with a history of childhood maltreatment', *Climacteric*, 25(2), pp. 203–207. doi: 10.1080/13697137.2021.1915270.
37. Carson, M. Y. and Thurston, R. C. (2019). 'Childhood abuse and vasomotor symptoms among midlife women',

Menopause, 26(10), pp. 1093–1099. doi: 10.1097/GME.0000000000001366.

38. ScienceDaily (2017). *Abuse accelerates puberty in children*, 17 March. Available at: https://www.sciencedaily.com/releases/2017/03/170328120237.htm
39. Open Access Government (2022). *Reproductive ageing in women affected by experience of abuse*, 16 February. Available at: https://www.openaccessgovernment.org/menopause-abuse/129764/# :~
40. National Center for Victims of Crime (no date). *Child Sexual Abuse Statistics*. Available at: https://victimsofcrime.org/child-sexual-abuse-statistics/
41. World Health Organization (2024). *Violence against women*, 25 March. Available at: https://www.who.int/news-room/fact-sheets/detail/violence-against-women
42. Strategic Market Research (2022). *Hormone Replacement Therapy Market Size & Trends, 2030*, January. Available at: https://www.strategicmarketresearch.com/market-report/hormone-replacement-therapy-market
43. Hickey, M., Hunter, M. S., Santoro, N. and Ussher, J. (2022). 'Normalising menopause', *BMJ*, e069369. doi: 10.1136/bmj-2021-069369.
44. Hoga, L., Rodolpho, J., Gonçalves, B. and Quirino, B. (2015). 'Women's experience of menopause: a systematic review of qualitative evidence', *JBI Database of Systematic Reviews and Implementation Reports*, 13(8), pp. 250–337. doi: 10.11124/JBISRIR-2015-1948.
45. Madden, S., St Pierre-Hansen, N., Kelly, L., Cromarty, H., Linkewich, B. and Payne, L. (2010). 'First Nations women's

knowledge of menopause: Experiences and perspectives', *PubMed Central*, September. Available at: https://www.ncbi.nlm.nih.gov/pmc/articles/PMC2939134/

46. Women's Health Network (2023). 'Menopause in different cultures', 28 February. Available at: https://www.womenshealthnetwork.com/menopause-and-perimenopause/menopause-in-different-cultures/ (last updated 8 Dec 2025)
47. Bagust, P. (2023). 'Māori wisdom on periods you didn't know you needed', *Grey Areas with Petra Bagust* [podcast]. Available at: https://open.spotify.com/episode/3R1kxfpqquMfh13hE41GM5?si=1ba7d12f24e74820
48. Young, C. (2022). 'Menopause the "Second spring"', *The Grove Chinese Medicine*, 24 August. Available at: https://thegroveclinic.com.au/blogs/news/menopause-the-second-spring# :~
49. Nappi, R. E., Kroll, R., Siddiqui, E., Stoykova, B., Rea, C., Gemmen, E. and Schultz, N. M. (2021). 'Global cross-sectional survey of women with vasomotor symptoms associated with menopause: prevalence and quality of life burden', *Menopause*, 28(8), pp. 875–882. doi: 10.1097/GME.0000000000001793.
50. Haines, C. J., Xing, S., Park, K., Holinka, C. F. and Ausmanas, M. K. (2005). 'Prevalence of menopausal symptoms in different ethnic groups of Asian women and responsiveness to therapy with three doses of conjugated estrogens/medroxyprogesterone acetate: The PanAsia menopause (PAM) study', *Maturitas*, 52(3–4), pp. 264–276. doi: 10.1016/j.maturitas.2005.03.012.

51. Hooper, L., Ryder, J., Kurzer, Lampe, J., Messina, M., Phipps, W. and Cassidy, A. (2009). 'Effects of soy protein and isoflavones on circulating hormone concentrations in pre and postmenopausal women: a systematic review and metaanalysis', *Human Reproduction Update*, 15(4), pp. 423–440. doi: 10.1093/humupd/dmp010.
52. Les Possédés et leurs mondes (2018). *Margaret Lock. Film 4. Research with Japanese Women on Menopause* [online video]. Available at: https://www.youtube.com/watch?v=nA3BwweXiIQ

Chapter 7

1. Aiello, S. (2021). 'Misogyny: The Driving Force of the Great European WitchHunts from the Fifteenth to Seventeenth Centuries', *Retrospect Journal*, 24 October. Available at: https://retrospectjournal.com/2021/10/24/misogyny-the-driving-force-of-the-great-european-witch-hunts-from-the-fifteenth-to-seventeenth-centuries/
2. Horstead, K. (2017). 'Witchcraft attacks are a symptom of ageism and sexism', *Age International Blog*, 27 October. Available at: https://blog.ageinternational.org.uk/witchcraft-abuse-symptomatic-ageism-sexism/
3. Roberts, Y. (2021). 'End femicide: 278 dead – the hidden scandal of older women killed by men', *The Guardian*, 7 March. Available at: https://www.theguardian.com/society/2021/mar/07/end-femicide-278-dead-the-hidden-scandal-of-older-women-killed-by-men

4. Femicide Census (2020). *Femicide Census 2020.* Available at: https://www.femicidecensus.org/wp-content/uploads/2022/02/010998-2020-Femicide-Report_V2.pdf
5. British Fertility Society (no date). *At what age does fertility begin to decrease?*. Available at: https://www.britishfertilitysociety.org.uk/fei/at-what-age-does-fertility-begin-to-decrease/
6. Dell'Amore, C. (2012). 'Women can make new eggs after all, StemCell study hints', *National Geographic*, 1 March. Available at: https://www.nationalgeographic.com/science/article/120229-women-health-ovaries-eggs-reproduction-science
7. ScienceDaily (2018). *Beluga whales and narwhals go through menopause*, 27 August. Available at: https://www.sciencedaily.com/releases/2018/08/180827080847.htm
8. Hood, M. (2016). 'Solving the evolutionary puzzle of menopause', *Phys.org*, 17 February. Available at: https://phys.org/news/2016-02-evolutionary-puzzle-menopause.html
9. Morton, R. A., Stone, J. R. and Singh, R. S. (2013). 'Mate choice and the origin of menopause', *PLOS Computational Biology*, 9(6), e1003092. doi: 10.1371/journal.pcbi.1003092.
10. Hawkes, K. and Smith, K. R. (2009). 'Brief communication: Evaluating grandmother effects', *American Journal of Physical Anthropology*, 140(1), pp. 173–176. doi: 10.1002/ajpa.21061.
11. Hawkes, K., O'Connell, J. F. and Jones, N. G. B. (1997). 'Hadza Women's time allocation, offspring provisioning, and the evolution of long postmenopausal life spans', *Current Anthropology*, 38(4), pp. 551–577. doi: 10.1086/204646.

12. Engelhardt, S. C., Bergeron, P., Gagnon, A., Dillon, L. and Pelletier, F. (2019). 'Using geographic distance as a potential proxy for help in the assessment of the grandmother hypothesis', Current Biology, 29(4), pp. 651–656.e3. doi: 10.1016/j.cub.2019.01.027.
13. Yong, E. (2015). 'Why killer whales go through menopause but elephants don't', *National Geographic*, 5 March. Available at: https://www.nationalgeographic.com/science/article/why-killer-whales-go-through-menopause-but-elephants-dont
14. Ruggeri, A. (2018). 'Do we really live longer than our ancestors?', *BBC Future*, 3 October. Available at: https://www.bbc.com/future/article/20181002-how-long-did-ancient-people-live-life-span-versus-longevity
15. Austad, S. N. and Bartke, A. (2015). 'Sex Differences in Longevity and in Responses to AntiAging Interventions: A MiniReview', *Gerontology*, 62(1), pp. 40–46. doi: 10.1159/000381472.
16. Kim, Y. J., Soto, M., Branigan, G. L., Rodgers, K. and Brinton, R. D. (2021). 'Association between menopausal hormone therapy and risk of neurodegenerative diseases: Implications for precision hormone therapy', *Alzheimer's & Dementia. Translational Research & Clinical Interventions*, 7(1). doi: 10.1002/trc2.12174.
17. Oxford Royale Academy (no date). *9 Scientists who didn't get the credit they deserved*. Available at: https://www.oxford-royale.com/articles/9-scientists-didnt-get-credit-deserved/

18. ScienceDaily (2014). *Significantly increased risk of stillbirth in males, study shows*, 29 November. Available at: https://www.sciencedaily.com/releases/2014/11/141127082348.htm
19. Zeitlin, J., SaurelCubizolles, M. J., de Mouzon, J., Rivera, L., Ancel, P. Y., Blondel, B. and Kaminski, M. (2002). 'Fetal sex and preterm birth: are males at greater risk?', *Human Reproduction*, 17(10), pp. 2762–2768. doi: 10.1093/humrep/17.10.2762.
20. Peacock, J. L., Marston, L., Marlow, N., Calvert, S. A. and Greenough, A. (2012). 'Neonatal and infant outcome in boys and girls born very prematurely', *Pediatric Research*, 71(3), pp. 305–310. doi: 10.1038/pr.2011.50.
21. Stower, H. (2014). 'Risky Y chromosome loss', *Nature Medicine*, 20(6), p. 594. doi: 10.1038/nm.3601.
22. Johns Hopkins Medicine (no date). *Surviving trauma: being a woman confers advantages*. Available at: https://www.hopkinsmedicine.org/news/media/releases/surviving_trauma_being_a_woman_confers_advantages
23. Office for National Statistics (2021). *Coronavirus (COVID19) and the different effects on men and women in the UK, March 2020 to February 2021*, 10 March. Available at: https://www.ons.gov.uk/peoplepopulationandcommunity/healthandsocialcare/conditionsanddiseases/articles/coronaviruscovid19andthedifferenteffectsonmenandwomenintheuk-march2020tofebruary2021/2021-03-10
24. Linde, P. (2020). 'Why is the coronavirus killing nearly twice as many men as women in Spain?', *EL PAÍS English*, 25 March. Available at: https://english.elpais.com/society/2020-03-25/

why-is-the-coronavirus-killing-nearly-twice-as-many-men-as-women-in-spain.html

25. Amanpour & Company, PBS (2020). *The hidden reason why men are more likely to die of COVID19* [online video]. Available at: https://www.pbs.org/wnet/amanpour-and-company/video/the-hidden-reason-why-men-are-more-likely-to-die-of-covid-19/
26. Eskes, T. and Haanen, C. (2007). 'Why do women live longer than men?', *European Journal of Obstetrics, Gynecology, and Reproductive Biology*, 133(2), pp. 126–133. doi: 10.1016/j.ejogrb.2007.01.006.
27. Viña, J., Borrás, C., Gambini, J., Sastre, J. and Pallardó, F. V. (2005). 'Why females live longer than males: Control of longevity by sex hormones', *Science of Aging Knowledge Environment*, 2005(23). doi: 10.1126/sageke.2005.23.pe17.
28. Min, K., Lee, C. and Park, H. (2012). 'The lifespan of Korean eunuchs', *Current Biology*, 22(18), R792–R793. doi: 10.1016/j.cub.2012.06.036.
29. Perls, T. T., Alpert, L. and Fretts, R. C. (1997). 'Middleaged mothers live longer', *Nature*, 389(6647), p. 133. doi: 10.1038/38148.
30. Pirkle, C. M., De Albuquerque Sousa, A. C. P., Alvarado, B. and Zunzunegui, M. (2014). 'Early maternal age at first birth is associated with chronic diseases and poor physical performance in older age: crosssectional analysis from the International Mobility in Aging Study', *BMC Public Health*, 14(1). doi: 10.1186/1471-2458-14-293.
31. MaxPlanckGesellschaft (2019). *How children influence the life expectancy of their parents*, 23 October. Available at:

https://www.mpg.de/14064449/children-influence-parents-life-expectancy

32. De Lange, A. G., Barth, C., Kaufmann, T., Anatürk, M., Suri, S., Ebmeier, K. P. and Westlye, L. T. (2020). 'The maternal brain: Regionspecific patterns of brain aging are traceable decades after childbirth', *Human Brain Mapping*, 41(16), pp. 4718–4729. doi: 10.1002/hbm.25152.
33. Nalewicki, J. (2023). 'Extreme longevity: The secret to living longer may be hiding with nuns . . . and jellyfish', *Live Science*, 30 March. Available at: https://www.livescience.com/the-secrets-to-extreme-longevity-may-be-hiding-with-nuns-and-jellyfish
34. AP (1995). 'A 120year lease on life outlasts apartment heir', *The New York Times*, 29 December. Available at: https://www.nytimes.com/1995/12/29/world/a-120-year-lease-on-life-outlasts-apartment-heir.html
35. Williams, S. (2019). 'Are women better ultraendurance athletes than men?', *BBC News*, 11 August. Available at: https://www.bbc.co.uk/news/world-49284389
36. GoettnerAbendroth, H. (no date). 'What is a Matriarchy?', *Modern Matriarchal Studies*. Available at: https://mmstudies.com/matriarchy/
37. Caputo, J., Pavalko, E. K. and Hardy, M. A. (2016). 'The LongTerm Effects of Caregiving on Women's Health and Mortality', *Journal of Marriage and Family*, 78(5), pp. 1382–1398. doi: 10.1111/jomf.12332.
38. Ziwica, K. (2020). 'It's time to properly consider the value of women's work', *Women's Agenda*, 16 April. Available at: https://womensagenda.com.au/latest/

if-you-thought-that-was-a-lot-of-money-consider-the-value-of-womens-work/

39. Walker, P. (2023). 'Gender pay gap for women in their 50s won't close before 2050, claims Labour', *The Guardian*, 28 May. Available at: https://www.theguardian.com/world/2023/may/28/gender-pay-gap-for-women-in-their-50s-wont-close-before-2050-claims-labour
40. Weaver, M. (2021). '"Witch" tweets reflect society's fear of older women, says Mary Beard', *The Guardian*, 9 February. Available at: https://www.theguardian.com/books/2021/feb/09/mary-beard-witch-tweets-reflect-society-fear-older-women

Index